Rapid Expert Consultations on the COVID-19 Pandemic

MARCH 14, 2020–APRIL 8, 2020

The National Academies of
SCIENCES · ENGINEERING · MEDICINE

THE NATIONAL ACADEMIES PRESS
Washington, DC
www.nap.edu

THE NATIONAL ACADEMIES PRESS   500 Fifth Street, NW   Washington, DC 20001

This activity was supported by a contract between the National Academy of Sciences and the U.S. Department of Health and Human Services' Office of the Assistant Secretary for Preparedness and Response (75A50120G00002). Any opinions, findings, conclusions, or recommendations expressed in this publication do not necessarily reflect the views of any organization or agency that provided support for the project.

International Standard Book Number-13: 978-0-309-67690-8
International Standard Book Number-10: 0-309-67690-8
Digital Object Identifier: https://doi.org/10.17226/25784

This publication is available from the National Academies Press, 500 Fifth Street, NW, Keck 360, Washington, DC 20001; (800) 624-6242 or (202) 334-3313; http://www.nap.edu.

Copyright 2020 by the National Academy of Sciences. All rights reserved.

Printed in the United States of America

Suggested citation: National Academies of Sciences, Engineering, and Medicine. 2020. *Rapid Expert Consultations for the COVID-19 Pandemic: March 14, 2020–April 8, 2020*. Washington, DC: The National Academies Press. https://doi.org/10.17226/25784.

The National Academies of
SCIENCES · ENGINEERING · MEDICINE

The **National Academy of Sciences** was established in 1863 by an Act of Congress, signed by President Lincoln, as a private, nongovernmental institution to advise the nation on issues related to science and technology. Members are elected by their peers for outstanding contributions to research. Dr. Marcia McNutt is president.

The **National Academy of Engineering** was established in 1964 under the charter of the National Academy of Sciences to bring the practices of engineering to advising the nation. Members are elected by their peers for extraordinary contributions to engineering. Dr. John L. Anderson is president.

The **National Academy of Medicine** (formerly the Institute of Medicine) was established in 1970 under the charter of the National Academy of Sciences to advise the nation on medical and health issues. Members are elected by their peers for distinguished contributions to medicine and health. Dr. Victor J. Dzau is president.

The three Academies work together as the **National Academies of Sciences, Engineering, and Medicine** to provide independent, objective analysis and advice to the nation and conduct other activities to solve complex problems and inform public policy decisions. The National Academies also encourage education and research, recognize outstanding contributions to knowledge, and increase public understanding in matters of science, engineering, and medicine.

Learn more about the National Academies of Sciences, Engineering, and Medicine at **www.nationalacademies.org**.

STANDING COMMITTEE ON EMERGING INFECTIOUS DISEASES AND 21ST CENTURY HEALTH THREATS

HARVEY V. FINEBERG (*Chair*), President, Gordon and Betty Moore Foundation
KRISTIAN G. ANDERSEN, Associate Professor, Immunology and Microbiology, The Scripps Research Institute
MARY T. BASSETT, FXB Professor of the Practice of Health and Human Rights, Harvard T.H. Chan School of Public Health
TREVOR BEDFORD, Associate Member, Vaccine and Infectious Disease Division, Fred Hutchinson Cancer Research Center
GEORGES C. BENJAMIN, Executive Director, American Public Health Association
RICHARD E. BESSER, President and Chief Executive Officer, Robert Wood Johnson Foundation
PETER DASZAK, President, EcoHealth Alliance
ELLEN P. EMBREY, Managing Partner, Stratitia Inc.
DIANE E. GRIFFIN, University Distinguished Service Professor and Alfred and Jill Sommer Chair of the W. Harry Feinstone Department of Molecular Microbiology and Immunology, Johns Hopkins Bloomberg School of Public Health
MARGARET A. HAMBURG, Foreign Secretary, National Academy of Medicine
JOHN L. HICK, Faculty Emergency Physician, Hennepin Healthcare and Professor of Emergency Medicine, University of Minnesota
KENT E. KESTER, Vice President and Head, Translational Science and Biomarkers, Sanofi Pasteur
PATRICIA A. KING, Professor of Law (Emeritus), Georgetown University Law Center
JONNA A. MAZET, Professor of Epidemiology and Disease Ecology, University of California, Davis, School of Veterinary Medicine
PHYLLIS D. MEADOWS, Senior Fellow, The Kresge Foundation
TARA O'TOOLE, Executive Vice President, In-Q-Tel
ALEXANDRA PHELAN, Assistant Professor, Center for Global Health Science and Security, Department of Microbiology and Immunology, Georgetown University
DAVID A. RELMAN, Thomas C. and Joan M. Merigan Professor in Medicine, Professor of Microbiology and Immunology, Stanford University
MARK S. SMOLINSKI, President, Ending Pandemics
DAVID R. WALT, Hansjörg Wyss Professor of Bioinspired Engineering, Harvard Medical School

Project Staff

LISA BROWN, Senior Program Officer
AUTUMN DOWNEY, Senior Program Officer
CAROLYN SHORE, Senior Program Officer
SCOTT WOLLEK, Senior Program Officer
AURELIA ATTAL-JUNCQUA, Associate Program Officer
EMMA FINE, Associate Program Officer
MICHAEL BERRIOS, Research Associate
BRIDGET BOREL, Administrative Assistant
JULIE PAVLIN, Senior Director, Board on Global Health
ANDREW M. POPE, Senior Director, Board on Health Sciences Policy

Acknowledgments

The National Academies of Sciences, Engineering and Medicine would like to acknowledge the contributions of the following subject-matter experts in developing these rapid expert consultations.

DONALD BERWICK, Institute for Healthcare Improvement
CARLOS DEL RIO, Emory Vaccine Center
BARUCH FISCHHOFF, Carnegie Mellon University
DAN HANFLING, In-Q-Tel
JAMES HODGE, Arizona State University
SUNDARESAN JAYARAMAN, Georgia Tech
MICHAEL OSTERHOLM, University of Minnesota
ED NARDEL, Harvard University
JENNIFER NUZZO, Johns Hopkins Bloomberg School of Public Health
RICHARD SERINO, Harvard T.H. Chan School of Public Health
BETH WEAVER, RESOLVE
MATTHEW WYNIA, University of Colorado Center for Bioethics and Humanities

The review of these rapid expert consultations was overseen by Bobbie Berkowitz, Columbia University School of Nursing; Ellen Wright Clayton, Vanderbilt University Medical Center; and Sue Curry, University of Iowa College of Public Health. They were responsible for making certain that independent examinations of these rapid expert consultations were carried out in accordance with the standards of the National Academies and that all review comments were carefully considered. Responsibility for the final content rests entirely with the authors and the National Academies.

Contents

Preface	xi
Rapid Expert Consultation on Severe Illness in Young Adults for the COVID-19 Pandemic (March 14, 2020)	1
Rapid Expert Consultation on SARS-CoV-2 Surface Stability and Incubation for the COVID-19 Pandemic (March 15, 2020)	5
Rapid Expert Consultation on Social Distancing for the COVID-19 Pandemic (March 19, 2020)	7
Rapid Expert Consultation on Data Elements and Systems Design for Modeling and Decision Making for the COVID-19 Pandemic (March 21, 2020)	11
Rapid Expert Consultation Update on SARS-CoV-2 Surface Stability and Incubation for the COVID-19 Pandemic (March 27, 2020)	15
Rapid Expert Consultation on Crisis Standards of Care for the COVID-19 Pandemic (March 28, 2020)	25
Rapid Expert Consultation on the Possibility of Bioaerosol Spread of SARS-CoV-2 for the COVID-19 Pandemic (April 1, 2020)	35
Rapid Expert Consultation on SARS-CoV-2 Survival in Relation to Temperature and Humidity and Potential for Seasonality for the COVID-19 Pandemic (April 7, 2020)	39

Rapid Expert Consultation on SARS-CoV-2 Laboratory Testing
for the COVID-19 Pandemic (April 8, 2020)   47

Rapid Expert Consultation on the Effectiveness of Fabric Masks
for the COVID-19 Pandemic (April 8, 2020)   55

Rapid Expert Consultation on SARS-CoV-2 Viral Shedding and
Antibody Response for the COVID-19 Pandemic (April 8, 2020)   63

Preface

The National Academies are a unique national resource. Their members represent the best in American science, engineering, and medicine. For more than a century, the National Academies have called upon their members and other experts to lend their knowledge and experience as volunteers in service to the nation. The National Academies have rightly been called objective, evidence-based, influential, and authoritative. In this instance, they have also proved to be quick.

The COVID-19 pandemic has demanded exceptional responses from many institutions, domestic and international, public and private. As the pandemic began to take hold in the United States, the White House Office of Science and Technology Policy, led by Dr. Kelvin Droegemeier, and the U.S. Department of Health and Human Services, in the person of Dr. Robert Kadlec, Assistant Secretary for Preparedness and Response, turned to the National Academies for expert advice. Presidents Marcia McNutt, John Anderson, and Victor Dzau responded by setting up the Standing Committee on Emerging Infectious Diseases and 21st Century Health Threats.

The standing committee held its first organizational meeting on Wednesday, March 11, 2020, and in consultation with the sponsors, prepared an initial list of scientific and technical questions that the COVID-19 pandemic posed. Sponsor assignments cascaded onto the committee, and the staff, members, and other experts responded with alacrity. The main work product in this phase has been the "rapid expert consultation," a written product prepared by the committee and subject to accelerated review by the quality assurance arm of the National Academies, its Report Review Committee.

As I write this, just 1 month after the initial, organizing meeting, the standing committee has produced 11 rapid expert consultations in addition to the initial listing of important issues, and it has organized one informal telephone consultation on behalf of the sponsors, a mechanism that allows government officials to tap even more rapidly into the expertise of the standing committee members and others. As we look ahead, we anticipate that the committee will begin to focus on intermediate-term questions, where the answers have a time constant measured in weeks to months rather than hours to days. We also expect to turn more regularly to the informal, telephonic consultations in which the sponsors can obtain expert input in a timely way and experts can be directly responsive to the most pressing questions.

With this expected transition in emphasis, this seems like an appropriate moment to collect the set of completed rapid expert consultations, assembled here. In this rapidly evolving pandemic, new knowledge emerges by the day, and these statements each represent a snapshot of what was known at a particular moment in time. While they were rapidly prepared, we also hope they represent sound, thoughtful, timely, and useful information for the decision makers who are shaping the nation's response to COVID-19.

I would like to express my appreciation to Drs. Droegemeier and Kadlec who placed their confidence in the National Academies, to the Academy presidents who established the standing committee, to the members of the committee and other experts who stepped up whenever asked, to the outside reviewers and Report Review Committee staff and leaders who moved briskly to improve the final products, and above all, to the exceptional standing committee staff who labored literally day and night to produce these documents.

As the National Academies contribute to policy decisions with objective, scientific, evidence-based guidance, these rapid expert consultations stand as testimony to an additional capability of the National Academies to act as swiftly as the current crisis demands.

Harvey V. Fineberg, M.D., Ph.D.
Chair
National Academies of Sciences, Engineering, and Medicine's Standing Committee
on Emerging Infectious Diseases and 21st Century Health Threats

Rapid Expert Consultation on Severe Illness in Young Adults for the COVID-19 Pandemic (March 14, 2020)

March 14, 2020

Kelvin Droegemeier, Ph.D.
Office of Science and Technology Policy
Executive Office of the President
Eisenhower Executive Office Building
1650 Pennsylvania Avenue, NW
Washington, DC 20504

Robert Kadlec, M.D.
Assistant Secretary for Preparedness and Response
200 Independence Avenue, SW
Washington, DC 20201

Dear Drs. Droegemeier and Kadlec:

Attached is a brief response to your question on whether reports of severe illness in younger adults in Italy may represent a genetic change to the virus. As explained in the note, the reports from Italy of severe illness in young adults may not represent a change in the pattern of susceptibility, as even the earliest reports from China indicated severe illness among young adults, though at a lower frequency than among older persons. At the present time, the genetic make up of the virus circulating in Italy appears to be the same as that found in other countries of Europe.

The enclosed document was prepared by staff of the National Academies of Sciences, Engineering, and Medicine based on input from Trevor Bedford, David Walt, and me.

My colleagues and I hope this input is helpful to you as you continue to guide the nation's response in this ongoing public health crisis.

Respectfully,
Harvey V. Fineberg, M.D., Ph.D.
Chair
Standing Committee on Emerging Infectious Diseases and 21st Century Health Threats

Recent reports from Italy describe severe illness requiring ventilatory support in younger adults without underlying comorbidities. At this time, there are not enough data to indicate whether these cases are a small fraction of a large number of infected young adults or represent a shift in the severity spectrum toward more severe disease in younger adults. Of note, China reported 12.0% (67/557) of patients 15-49 years of age developed severe illness (compared to 28.8% [44/153] in those ≥65 years),[1] so severe illness in young adults has not been an uncommon occurrence from the start of the pandemic.[2] Unofficial reports from the outbreak in the state of Washington similarly note the occurrence of severe illness in young adults.

A determination of any change in the incidence or severity spectrum of illness in different segments of the population requires a systematic analysis of longitudinal data, currently unavailable. Obtaining these data through the tracking of natural patient histories and outcomes is an important component of managing the epidemic. This analysis would produce updated calculations of risk factors by age group and tracking of any changes over time. We need to be prepared to routinely collect and share these data as the epidemic progresses in the United States.

If changes in risk factor by age group were to occur, this could potentially be a result of mutations in the circulating virus. On genomic epidemiologic analysis, the Italian outbreak is primarily driven by the "Lombardy clade" or "A2."[3] This clade has a P314L mutation in ORF1b and also R203K and G204R in N. However, this same virus is distributed widely throughout Europe, and there are not enough data reported from other European countries to conclude whether the Italian experience is atypical. The epidemic expanded rapidly in Italy prior to an increase in cases in other European countries. If Italy is reporting an increase in severity and deaths among young adults compared to other European countries, this could be due to the stage of the epidemic, health system shortcomings, or different reporting methods rather than virus evolution.

---

[1] Guan et al. 2020. Clinical characteristics of coronavirus disease 2019 in China. *New England Journal of Medicine*. DOI: 10.1056/NEJMoa2002032.

[2] The manuscript defines "severe" as per the American Thoracic Society guidelines and not all severe cases may have required mechanical ventilation. In addition, the manuscript does not delineate by age group how many severe cases had underlying illnesses (38.7% of severe cases overall had a coexisting disorder). Metlay et al. 2019. Diagnosis and treatment of adults with community-acquired pneumonia: An official clinical practice guideline of the American Thoracic Society and Infectious Diseases Society of America. *American Journal of Respiratory and Critical Care Medicine* 200(7):e45-e67. DOI: 10.1164/rccm.201908-1581ST.

[3] See https://nextstrain.org/ncov?branchLabel=aa&label=clade:A2&m=div.

Although COVID-19 typically has caused higher rates of severe illness and mortality in older populations and those with underlying illnesses, it is important not to downplay the potential seriousness of this infection in younger age groups. While data are gathered and analyzed, messaging should stress that everyone should be concerned about COVID-19 and take appropriate steps to protect their health, the health of their loved ones and neighbors, and the health of the public at large.

Rapid Expert Consultation on SARS-CoV-2 Surface Stability and Incubation for the COVID-19 Pandemic (March 15, 2020)

March 15, 2020

Kelvin Droegemeier, Ph.D.
Office of Science and Technology Policy
Executive Office of the President
Eisenhower Executive Office Building
1650 Pennsylvania Avenue, NW
Washington, DC 20504

Dear Dr. Droegemeier:

You requested immediate feedback on two crucial questions. The following expert members of the Standing Committee on Emerging Infectious Diseases and 21st Century Health Threats were involved in preparing this document: Kent Kester, David Relman, David Walt, and me. Ellen Wright Clayton, Vanderbilt University, reviewed this document.

Question 1: Survival of virus on surfaces. One of the most thorough and informative studies is just now under consideration for publication and has not undergone full peer review. The investigators are a highly reputable group, and we can expect that their study was carefully conducted. They tested both the current coronavirus (SARS-CoV-2) and the original SARS virus (SARS-CoV-1). Results were similar for both viruses. They tested the viability (survival) of both viruses after controlled aerosolization and on a variety of surfaces. The aerosol (particles smaller than 5 microns that can float in the air) showed viral detection up to 3 hours post aerosolization. Following surface contamination, SARS-CoV-2 could be detected up to 4 hours on copper, up to 24 hours on cardboard and up to 2-3 days on plastic and on stainless steel. These results are consistent with the plausibility of both aerosol and surface (fomite) transmission of SARS-CoV-2. The difference in survival on copper (4 hours) and on stainless steel (2-3 days) is noteworthy. Note that this study excludes what is probably the most common route of spread, direct droplet transmission by cough or sneeze, or even exhalation by an infected person. Additionally, the members of the standing committee identified above note that the National Biodefense Analysis and Countermeasures Center (NBACC) is conducting environmental survival studies of SARS-CoV-2 and their results should be taken into account.

Question 2: Incubation period (time between exposure and onset of symptoms). Note that it is possible for viral shedding to begin prior to the onset of symptoms. Also, we are not considering here the question of how long viral shedding can continue in someone who has been infected. Rather, as we understand it, the question here pertains to the appropriate period of quarantine for an exposed individual. One of the more informative reports on incubation period studied 181 patients in China who had identifiable dates of exposure and of symptom onset.[1] In this study, the mean incubation period was estimated to be 5.1 days (95% confidence interval 4.5 to 5.8 days) and 97.5% of those who develop symptoms will do so within 11.5 days (95% confidence interval 8.2 to 15.6 days) of exposure. These estimates imply that only about 1% of cases (101/10,000) will develop symptoms following 14 days after exposure. Shortening quarantine to fewer than 14 days would increase the fraction who were still to develop symptoms. Note that Lauer et al. acknowledged that publicly reported cases may overrepresent severe cases, the incubation period for which may differ from that of mild cases.

Respectfully,
Harvey V. Fineberg, M.D., Ph.D.
Chair
Standing Committee on Emerging Infectious Diseases and 21st Century Health Threats

---

[1] Lauer et al. 2020. The incubation period of coronavirus disease 2019 (COVID-19) from publicly reported confirmed cases: Estimation and application free. *Annals of Internal Medicine*. DOI: 10.7326/M20-0504.

Rapid Expert Consultation on Social Distancing for the COVID-19 Pandemic (March 19, 2020)

March 19, 2020

Kelvin Droegemeier, Ph.D.
Office of Science and Technology Policy
Executive Office of the President
Eisenhower Executive Office Building
1650 Pennsylvania Avenue, NW
Washington, DC 20504

Dear Dr. Droegemeier:

This letter responds to your question about evidence on the effectiveness and costs of social distancing measures in contending with COVID-19.

Respiratory viruses are transmitted from person to person via air droplet (talk, sneeze, cough), suspended droplet nuclei (<5 microns diameter; sneeze, cough), and surface fomites (touch contaminated surface and then touch mucous membrane in eye, nose, mouth). Social distancing measures are based on the idea of interrupting these forms of transmission by separating infected and uninfected persons. In the absence of a vaccine or effective prophylactic agents, social distancing is the principal tool available to blunt the force of an epidemic.[1]

---

[1] Qualls et al. 2017. Community mitigation guidelines to prevent pandemic influenza—United States, 2017. *Morbidity and Mortality Weekly Report—Recommendations and Reports* 66(1):1-32. DOI: 10.15585/mmwr.rr6601a1.

This response was prepared by staff of the National Academies of Sciences, Engineering, and Medicine based on input from Alexandra Phelan and me. Ned Calonge, The Colorado Trust; Sue Curry, University of Iowa; and Steven Teutsch, University of California, Los Angeles, reviewed this document, and Ellen Wright Clayton, Vanderbilt University, approved the document on behalf of the Report Review Committee. The attached materials summarize evidence bearing on the effectiveness of social distancing measures, and they demonstrate that social distancing measures are effective. However, their effectiveness depends on such factors as early implementation and compliance.

Most of these studies are based on past experience with influenza. Some are empirical studies of the experience in different places that employed varying degrees of social separation during the great influenza pandemic of 1918-1919. Others are modeling exercises using available data and certain assumptions about relevant characteristics of an infection, such as the basic reproductive number, degree of mixing, and fraction of susceptible individuals. In general, these studies support the value of social distancing in reducing the amount of illness and death and in spreading the onset of illness over a longer time period ("flattening the curve"), which makes clinical management more feasible. For example, one study of 34 U.S. cities during the 1918-1919 influenza pandemic found that those communities that implemented social distancing measures earlier experienced greater delays in reaching peak mortality, lower peak mortality rates, and lower total mortality.[2]

In interpreting these data, it is important to note that "social distancing" can cover a wide range of community-based interventions, from closing schools and workplaces to eliminating mass public events to wearing face masks, and it is not always clear exactly which intervention is contributing what degree to the differential outcomes. Also important in the current context are differences between influenza and SARS-CoV-2 in such key attributes as transmission rate, incubation period, uncertainty regarding children as vectors, and pre-existing immunity in the population.

In general, studies based on historical data and on modeling both indicate that social distancing interventions are more effective when instituted early in the course of an epidemic.[3,4]

Only a handful of studies consider cost-effectiveness of this class of interventions, and many of them include consideration of pharmaceutical interventions such as antiviral treatments and vaccination strategies that are not currently available for this

---

[2] Markel et al. 2007. Nonpharmaceutical interventions implemented by US cities during the 1918-1919 influenza pandemic. *JAMA* 298(6):644-654. DOI: 10.1001/jama.298.6.644.

[3] Hatchett et al. 2007. Public health interventions and epidemic intensity during the 1918 influenza pandemic. *PNAS* 104(18):7582-7587. https://doi.org/10.1073/pnas.0610941104.

[4] Halloran et al. 2008. Modeling targeted layered containment of an influenza pandemic in the United States. *PNAS* 105(12):4639-4644. DOI: 10.1073/pnas.0706849105.

pandemic.[5,6,7,8] In general, these studies do not fully incorporate all social and economic costs that attend to such interventions as the cancellation of travel and the suspension of many businesses. They are not updated to today's economic and social circumstances, and the comparison to "benefits" relate to the burden of influenza, not SARS-CoV-2. Therefore, they do not have much to reveal about the cost or cost-effectiveness of today's interventions in the current pandemic.

More pertinent to decision making today about COVID-19 is the experience of other countries where the pandemic preceded outbreaks in the United States.

In an informative analysis, for example, Wang et al. evaluated the impact of social distancing and case finding and isolation of patients over three phases of the epidemic in Wuhan, China.[9] Prior to introducing any of these measures, the basic reproductive number was estimated to be 3.86 (95% credible interval 3.74 to 3.97). This period, from December 8, 2019, to January 23, 2020, was marked by an exponential growth in new cases. From January 23, 2020, to February 2, 2020, the following social distancing measures were implemented: home quarantine for suspected cases, cordon sanitaire, suspension of public transportation, closure of entertainment venues and public spaces, compulsory wearing of face masks, mandated personal hygiene, and body temperature self-monitoring. During this period, the reproductive number fell to 1.26, a substantial improvement, but still above the level of 1.0 that sustains spread. From February 2, 2020, and on, cordon sanitaire, suspension of public transportation, closure of entertainment venues and public spaces continued, and the following measures were also implemented: centralized isolation in designated hospitals for cases; mobile-cabin hospitals, schools, and hotels for exposed and possible cases; universal and strict stay-at-home policy for all residents unless permitted; widespread temperature and symptom monitoring; and universal screening and reporting. With these added measures the basic reproductive number fell to 0.32, and the epidemic subsided. The interventions were estimated to prevent 94.5% (93.7 to 95.2%) of infections until February 18.

A recent modeling exercise reported from Imperial College London[10] examined the effectiveness of different social distancing strategies to mitigate or suppress the force of the epidemic in the United Kingdom and the United States. The overall conclusion is that population-wide social distancing in combination with home isolation of cases, quarantine of exposed individuals, and school and university closure could reduce the

---

[5] Milne et al. 2013. The cost effectiveness of pandemic influenza interventions: A pandemic severity based analysis. *PLOS ONE* 8(4):e61504. DOI: 10.1371/journal.pone.0061504.

[6] Pasquini-Descomps et al. 2017. Value for money in H1N1 influenza: A systematic review of the cost-effectiveness of pandemic interventions. *Value in Health* 20(6):819-827. DOI: 10.1016/j.jval.2016.05.005.

[7] Pérez Velasco et al. 2017. Systematic review of economic evaluations of preparedness strategies and interventions against influenza pandemics. *PLOS ONE* 7(2):e30333. DOI: 10.1371/journal.pone.0030333.

[8] Perlroth et al. 2010. Health outcomes and costs of community mitigation strategies for an influenza pandemic in the United States. *Clinical Infectious Diseases* 50(2):165-174. DOI: 10.1086/649867.

[9] Wang et al. 2020. Evolving epidemiology and impact of non-pharmaceutical interventions on the outbreak of coronavirus disease 2019 in Wuhan, China. *medRxiv*. https://doi.org/10.1101/2020.03.03.20030593.

[10] Ferguson et al. 2020. Impact of non-pharmaceutical interventions (NPIs) to reduce COVID-19 mortality and healthcare demand. Imperial College London (16-03-2020). DOI: https://doi.org/10.25561/77482.

incidence of new cases (suppress) and not merely slow the rise (mitigate). However, to avoid the re-emergence of the disease, their models indicate these interventions would need to be maintained until an effective vaccine is developed and deployed, and this could take 18 months or longer. The authors stress uncertainty in estimates of transmissibility and effectiveness of interventions. They acknowledge the practical possibility of shorter-term interventions and variation across geographies depending on the local stage of the outbreak. Their analysis suggests that a 3-month period of intervention, stressing social distancing of vulnerable (older or chronically ill) populations in combination with other measures could reduce deaths in half and peak health care demand by two-thirds. At the same time, half-measures, such as case isolation and social distancing of the elderly only (rather than the entire population), could lead to an epidemic that overwhelms hospital surge capacity and, they project, could cause more than 1 million deaths in the United States.

Anecdotally, Singapore, which after the experience of the SARS outbreak in 2002 refined its capacity for intensive detection, isolation of cases, contact tracing, and quarantine of exposed individuals, has managed to suppress the SARS-CoV-2 epidemic without resorting as yet to closing schools and workplaces. These results are possible only with the availability of widespread diagnostic testing. The continued influx of new cases, probably related to travel, creates an ongoing challenge for the public health authorities there.

In the United States, we are embarked on a natural experiment where different communities will likely enact different levels and timing of social distancing relative to the local phase of the epidemic. Experience in other countries during the current COVID-19 pandemic shows the value of widely available diagnostic testing to guide the response. If our nation mounts a coordinated effort to detect and monitor disease incidence and tracks the control measures that are being implemented in each community, compliance rates, and other relevant data, we can better inform decisions about when social distancing measures may be withdrawn and in what circumstances they may need to be reinstated or enlarged. Judgments about when to suspend which social distancing measures will be critical and should involve discussions with public health experts, mathematical modelers, economists, and social and behavioral scientists. Decision makers will be greatly aided by ongoing data collection and disease monitoring.

My colleagues and I hope this rapid expert consultation is helpful to you as you continue to guide the nation's response in this ongoing public health crisis.

Respectfully,
Harvey V. Fineberg, M.D., Ph.D.
Chair
Standing Committee on Emerging Infectious Diseases and 21st Century Health Threats

Rapid Expert Consultation on Data Elements and Systems Design for Modeling and Decision Making for the COVID-19 Pandemic (March 21, 2020)

March 21, 2020

Kelvin Droegemeier, Ph.D.
Office of Science and Technology Policy
Executive Office of the President
Eisenhower Executive Office Building
1650 Pennsylvania Avenue, NW
Washington, DC 20504

Dear Dr. Droegemeier:

This letter responds to your question about necessary data elements, sources of data, gaps in collection, and suggestions for data system design and integration to improve modeling and decision making for COVID-19.

We enumerate eight basic points of perspective on the question you posed.

1. Utilizing existing databases and focusing on accessibility, usability, interoperability, and scalability will lead more rapidly to functional data systems than attempting to build systems from scratch.
2. It is better to start with basic functions that cover only the fundamental needs for viral tracking, epidemic monitoring and modeling, clinical management, resource deployment, and public communication.
3. Depending on the intended range of users and uses, the relevant data may include disease surveillance, longitudinal clinical health information, human genomic data, viral genomic data, medical supplies and logistics, and sociodemographic and behavioral data.

4. Choices about system architecture, design elements, and desired outputs are best made in concert with choices of software and system platforms.
5. Integration will be a challenge across public and private sources; clinical care and public health; and local, state, and national levels.
6. Anticipate the need to fill gaps in currently available data systems, including in public health information currently collected by individual states and local authorities.[1]
7. Attempt to design so as to reduce tradeoffs across accessibility and security, ease of use and comprehensiveness, and local utility and scalability.
8. Clarity about the prospective users and purposes of the system will greatly aid making sensible design choices and tradeoffs. A data system intended to serve all needs for everyone is liable to end up satisfying no one's basic needs.

We can use data systems to (1) determine community spread and impact; (2) monitor the clinical spectrum of illness to include response to treatment; and (3) provide accurate, up-to-date information to feed into models to forecast disease rates and subsequent clinical and logistical needs and the effectiveness of mitigation plans. All three contribute to the public health and clinical and logistical response to an epidemic.

Useful community patient data precede specific diagnoses of a COVID-19 infection. Available systems illustrate the richness of current data gathering and the opportunity for integration and interoperability. At a syndromic level (symptoms and signs prior to a final diagnosis), the Centers for Disease Control and Prevention's (CDC's) National Syndromic Surveillance Program (NSSP) collects emergency room visit data across the United States, including the reason for the visit and, as appropriate, a diagnosis.[2] Collaborating commercial laboratories are providing SARS-CoV-2 testing and results into the NSSP in a near-real-time basis. In addition, using traditional influenza surveillance programs that track influenza-like symptoms along with confirmed laboratory tests (CDC's FluView), the NSSP is comparing emergency room symptoms with test results to assess divergence, which could indicate COVID-19 infections in those communities. The Flu Near You program out of HealthMap and the American Public Health Association is a participatory surveillance program that allows the public to report symptoms by geographic location. This program is being relaunched as a COVID Near You program that can also evaluate human behaviors along with health status. These programs illustrate the richness of existing data-gathering systems, to include smartphone technology and social media outreach, and an opportunity to take fuller advantage of the complementary information they provide.

Complete and accurate clinical data may include exposure information, reliable markers of disease progression and severity, important comorbidities such as diabetes and heart and lung disease, relevant conditions such as pregnancy (and obstetric outcomes), treatment protocols, geo-locations, and mortality. These data ideally will come from trusted sources. Most hospitals use electronic data records that can differ across

---

[1] Local public health authorities can invoke section 45 CFR 164.512(b) of the Health Insurance Portability and Accountability Act (HIPAA) to obtain protected health information without authorization in order to prevent or control COVID-19.

[2] For additional information on the NSSP, see https://www.cdc.gov/nssp/images/nsspinfo/Final_NSSP-Infographic.pdf.

institutions, localities, and states. Deploying a system of systems, it may be possible to consolidate clinical data and augment these programs to include additional elements. The use of natural language processing on narrative notes and sharing the analysis through a distributed query architecture has been accomplished regionally for clinical research and could be expanded. Programs such as the Shared Health Research Information Network,[3] the Patient-Centered Outcomes Research Institute's Clinical Data Research Network[4] and the Observational Health Data Sciences and Informatics' Observational Medical Outcomes Partnership Common Data Model[5] all support interoperability of core datasets. Starting with basic descriptive statistics of patients and expanding as more data and techniques are available can assist with triage and identify important biological themes.

Whether for a known infectious pathogen or a novel one, the ability to model the pathogenesis, transmission, effective control strategies, and spread of a disease can provide crucial information to those needing to make decisions about the distribution of limited resources. An example of a successful collaborative effort is the Models of Infectious Disease Agent Study (MIDAS).[6] This effort, funded by the National Institute of General Medical Sciences at the National Institutes of Health, is a global network of research scientists and practitioners who develop and use computational, statistical, and mathematical models to understand infectious disease dynamics. MIDAS has an online portal to share data and information regarding the COVID-19 pandemic and could be used as a resource for decision makers. To assist with forecasting disease progression and identifying important clinical markers before we obtain more data on COVID-19 in the United States, data from other countries, such as the daily number of hospitalizations, intensive care admissions, ventilator use, and deaths, can be used in forecasting expected epidemic progression and assist with clinical care decisions.

Assessing the capacity of medical facilities to provide intensive care to those in need will facilitate the allocation of ICU beds and ventilators. Programs at local and regional levels currently monitor the availability of hospital beds and other resources, and expanding these programs would provide a national view of areas most in need. Tracking mortality from disease in relation to resources can aid in the interpretation of fatality rates and inform future pandemic preparedness.

Current estimates surrounding the use of social interventions can be examined, evaluated, and adjusted using social data. The number of contacts being isolated and monitored and facility closings by state and region can be monitored along with de-identified social media postings that correlate with behaviors. Some insight into the impact of isolation and closings of schools, worksites, and volunteer programs can also be monitored through social media and voluntary reporting.

Knowing how a virus mutates as it moves through a population is vital to understanding possible changes in disease severity or transmissibility, amenity to diagnosis, and responsiveness to vaccine. This is an issue of global interest and will involve

---

[3] McMurry et al. 2013. SHRINE: Enabling nationally scalable multi-site disease studies. *PLOS ONE* 8(3):e55811. DOI: 10.1371/journal.pone.0055811.

[4] See https://www.pcori.org/research-results/pcornet%C2%AE-national-patient-centered-clinical-research-network.

[5] See https://www.ohdsi.org/data-standardization/the-common-data-model.

[6] See https://midasnetwork.us.

scientists from many parts of the world. International data sharing and enlisting tech companies that have the ability to provide data acquisition and processing would be important components of a comprehensive data system.

Moving forward, data collection tools can be designed to improve consolidation and sharing. For basic public health data, working with organizations that bring together local and state health departments (such as the Association of State and Territorial Health Officials [ASTHO], the National Association of County & City Health Officials [NACCHO], and the Council of State and Territorial Epidemiologists [CSTE]) would be a good starting point to ensure participation from across the public health community.

By following these principles, we believe it will be possible to rapidly assemble data systems that can inform decisions on managing the epidemic.

This response was prepared by staff of the National Academies of Sciences, Engineering, and Medicine based on input from Georges Benjamin, Ellen Embrey, Peggy Hamburg, Kent Kester, Patricia King, Jonna Mazet, Alexandra Phelan, Mark Smolinksi, David Walt, and me. Ned Calonge, The Colorado Trust; Marie Griffin and Kevin Johnson, Vanderbilt University Medical Center; Sandro Galea, Boston University; and Isaac Kohane, Harvard Medical School, reviewed this document, and Ellen Wright Clayton, Vanderbilt University, approved the document as monitor on behalf of the Report Review Committee.

Should you desire more substantive and detailed recommendations on system design and content, we would be happy to take this up over a suitable time frame. My colleagues and I hope this input is helpful to you as you continue to guide the nation's response in this ongoing public health crisis.

Respectfully,
Harvey V. Fineberg, M.D., Ph.D.
Chair
Standing Committee on Emerging Infectious Diseases and 21st Century Health Threats

Rapid Expert Consultation Update on SARS-CoV-2 Surface Stability and Incubation for the COVID-19 Pandemic (March 27, 2020)

March 27, 2020

Kelvin Droegemeier, Ph.D.
Office of Science and Technology Policy
Executive Office of the President
Eisenhower Executive Office Building
1650 Pennsylvania Avenue, NW
Washington, DC 20504

Dear Dr. Droegemeier:

You requested an update and elaboration on our previous rapid expert consultation dated March 15, concerning issues of virus survival on surfaces and in the air, and virus/disease incubation period. Here, we provide an update and elaboration on these issues, as well as some caveats about the work performed so far and as yet unmet needs. As with other questions and issues related to SARS-CoV-2 and COVID-19, work on these two topics is proceeding at a rapid pace at many locations across the globe. Consequently, aspects of this update may rapidly be superseded by new data.

This rapid expert consultation is organized by question and summarizes published and unpublished studies that were deemed most useful, as well as personal communications with experts (cited below). We have selected studies that are most relevant and critical, rather than attempting to be comprehensive. For each of the questions, data are presented for experimental studies and natural history studies, followed by comments on caveats and unmet needs.

This document was prepared by me with support from staff of the National Academies of Sciences, Engineering, and Medicine. Harvey Fineberg approved this document as chair of the Standing Committee on Emerging Infectious Diseases and 21st Century Health Threats. The following individuals served as reviewers: Kathryn Edwards, Vanderbilt University Medical Center; James LeDuc, University of Texas Medical Branch; and Linsey Marr, Virginia Tech. Ellen Wright Clayton, Vanderbilt University, and Susan Curry, University of Iowa, served as arbiters of this review on behalf of the National Academies' Report Review Committee and their Health and Medicine Division.

QUESTION 1: ENVIRONMENTAL SURVIVAL

In general, there are two basic approaches to study this issue: (A) experimental studies, typically involving the deliberate dissemination of a laboratory-propagated virus under controlled environmental conditions and subsequent sampling; and (B) natural history studies, typically involving the characterization of environments naturally contaminated by a virus, such as hospital rooms recently occupied by patients. Each approach has strengths and weaknesses: with experimental studies there is control over important parameters, but almost always the conditions fail to adequately mimic those of the natural setting; with natural history studies, the conditions are relevant and reflect the real world, but there is typically little control of environmental conditions and potentially confounding factors. Since March 15, there have been advances with studies of each type.

A. Experimental Studies

In a recent study from Hong Kong, Chin et al. examined the stability (using viral culture) of SARS-CoV-2 as a function of temperature, type of surface, and following the use of disinfectants.[1] With respect to temperature, using a starting suspension of 6.7 log $TCID_{50}$/ml in virus transport medium,[2] at 4°C there was only a 0.6-log unit reduction at the end of 14 days of incubation in this medium; at 22°C, a 3-log unit reduction after 7 days, and no detection at 14 days; and at 37°C, a 3-log unit reduction after 1 day and no virus detected afterward. No virus was detected after 30 minutes at 56°C or after 5 minutes at 70°C. With respect to survival on surfaces using a 5 µL droplet of virus culture at 7.8 log $TCID_{50}$/ml, no infectious virus was recovered from printing and tissue paper after 3 hours; no infectious virus was detected on cloth after 2 days or on stainless steel after 7 days. However, on the outside of a surgical mask, 0.1% of the original inoculum was detected on day 7. The persistence of infectious virus on personal protective equipment (PPE) is concerning and warrants additional study to inform guidance for health care workers. Such studies should also examine the effects of various treatments that might be used to disinfect PPE when they cannot be discarded after single use.

Chad Roy from the Tulane University National Primate Research Center shared via telephone some preliminary results of dynamic aerosol stability experiments with SARS-CoV-2 conducted over the past several weeks at the Infectious Disease

---

[1] Chin et al. 2020. Stability of SARS-CoV-2 in different environmental conditions. https://www.medrxiv.org/content/10.1101/2020.03.15.20036673v1.full.pdf (accessed March 24, 2020).

[2] $TCID_{50}$ is the Median Tissue Culture Infectious Dose.

Aerobiology Core program at Tulane.[3] His group generated an aerosol with a fairly uniform distribution of 2 micron particles, using virus grown in DMEM tissue culture (TC) medium and suspended in a rotating drum at an ambient temperature of ~23ºC and ~50% humidity. The aerosol was sampled longitudinally for up to 16 hours, and the virus was assessed for viability by growth (enumeration of plaque forming units [PFUs]) and morphology (electron microscopy). He reports surprisingly that SARS-CoV-2 has a longer half-life under these conditions than influenza virus, SARS-CoV-1, monkeypox virus, and *Mycobacterium tuberculosis*. He is still waiting for some growth results, but expects to post a manuscript describing these findings to bioRxiv on March 27. This result is also concerning, but is quite preliminary; importantly, the details have not yet been shared.

George Korch and Mike Hevey from the National Biodefense Analysis and Countermeasures Center (NBACC), which was created by the U.S. Department of Homeland Security, shared their plans for an extensive series of experiments on SARS-CoV-2 environmental survival.[4] Because they have shared these plans with the White House Coronavirus Task Force, only a few observations are provided here. The NBACC is well suited for the kinds of studies it has planned, and the scope and relevance are noteworthy. In particular, it plans to create simulated infected body fluids, including saliva and lower respiratory secretions. It plans to test simulated solar radiation on virus survival, which is important. It also has already examined a wider range of relative humidity and temperature than some other groups, which is again, important. And they will compare RNA semi-quantitative measurements with viral growth (PFUs) on samples from all conditions, which is critical.

At Rocky Mountain Laboratories (RML), part of the National Institutes of Health, current studies include the effect of temperature and humidity on virus stability; virus stability in human body fluids, including urine and feces; and the effectiveness of decontamination procedures for PPE, including N95 respirators.[5]

As follow-up, the study by van Doremalen et al. mentioned in our rapid expert consultation on March 15, which was at that time an unpublished preprint, has since been published by the *New England Journal of Medicine*.[6]

B. Natural History Studies

In a recent published study from Singapore, Ong et al. sampled environmental surfaces at 26 sites in each of 3 SARS-CoV-2 patient isolation rooms, as well as PPE worn by physicians exiting patient rooms and air in the patient rooms and anterooms.[7] All samples were tested using reverse transcriptase-polymerase chain reaction (RT-PCR).

---

[3] Personal communication, Chad Roy, Tulane University National Primate Research Center, March 24, 2020.

[4] Personal communication, George Korch and Mike Hevey, National Biodefense Analysis and Countermeasures Center, March 24, 2020.

[5] Personal communication, Vincent Munster, Rocky Mountain Laboratories, March 24, 2020.

[6] van Doremalen et al. 2020. Aerosol and surface stability of SARS-CoV-2 as compared with SARS-CoV-1. *New England Journal of Medicine*. DOI: 10.1056/NEJMc2004973.

[7] Ong et al. 2020. Air, surface environmental, and personal protective equipment contaminated by severe acute respiratory syndrome coronavirus 2 (SARS-CoV-2) from a symptomatic patient. *JAMA*. https://jamanetwork.com/journals/jama/fullarticle/2762692 (accessed March 24, 2020).

There were no efforts to assess virus viability. Patient A's room was sampled on days 4 and 10 of illness while the patient was still symptomatic after routine cleaning. All samples were negative. Patient B was symptomatic on day 8 and asymptomatic on day 11 of illness; samples taken on these 2 days after routine cleaning were negative. Samples collected from Patient C's room before routine cleaning had positive results at 13 (87%) of 15 room sites (including air outlet fans) and 3 (60%) of 5 toilet sites (toilet bowl, sink, and door handle). Anteroom and corridor samples were negative. Patient C had upper respiratory tract involvement with no pneumonia and had 2 positive stool samples for SARS-CoV-2 on RT-PCR, despite not having diarrhea. Only 1 PPE swab, from the surface of a shoe front, was positive. All other PPE swabs were negative. All air samples were negative. However, the lack of detection of the virus in air samples does not necessarily contradict the finding of the virus on the air outlet fan in Patient C's room, which presumably deposited from air onto the surface of the fan. There are at least three explanations for the negative findings in air: (1) a high ventilation rate of the room would dilute concentrations to a level that would be difficult to detect except with a large volume of air; (2) the sample volume was only a fraction of the total room volume; and (3) the air outlets were located above the head of the bed, and it is likely that any virus released into air would be transported directly upward to the outlet, so an air sampler would need to intersect this pathway to optimize chances of detection. Again, it is important to underscore that samples from the two surface-negative rooms were collected <u>after</u> the rooms had been cleaned.

In a recent unpublished study from Changchun, China, Jiang et al. collected 158 environmental surface and air samples from inside and near isolation wards where persons under investigation (PUIs) and known infected patients were housed.[8] Samples were collected just before daily cleaning procedures. Only 2 of the 158 samples were RT-PCR-positive: one from surfaces at a nursing station, and the other from an air sample from the room of an intensive care patient.

The Centers for Disease Control and Prevention (CDC) Cruise Ship Environmental Investigation Team mentioned in the CDC's *Morbidity and Mortality Weekly Report* (*MMWR*) on March 23, 2020, the results of environmental sample analysis from the Diamond Princess cruise ship.[9] In total, 601 samples were collected and tested, of which 58 were positive (9.7%) by RT-PCR. According to the Discussion, "SARS-CoV-2 RNA was identified on a variety of surfaces in cabins of both symptomatic and asymptomatic infected passengers up to 17 days after cabins were vacated on the Diamond Princess but before disinfection procedures had been conducted (Takuya Yamagishi, National Institute of Infectious Diseases, personal communication, 2020). Although these data cannot be used to determine whether transmission occurred from contaminated surfaces, further study of fomite transmission of SARS-CoV-2 aboard cruise ships is warranted."

Santarpia et al. recently completed a study (as yet unpublished and not yet posted on a preprint server) of air and surface samples from 11 isolation rooms at the University

---

[8] Jiang et al. 2020. Clinical data on hospital environmental hygiene monitoring and medical staffs protection during the coronavirus disease 2019 outbreak. https://www.medrxiv.org/content/10.1101/2020.02.25.20028043v2.full.pdf (accessed March 25, 2020).

[9] Moriarty et al. 2020. Public health responses to COVID-19 outbreaks on cruise ships—worldwide, February–March 2020. *Morbidity and Mortality Weekly Report* 69(12):347-352. http://dx.doi.org/10.15585/mmwr.mm6912e3.

of Nebraska Medical Center that were used to care for SARS-CoV-2 patients.[10] Samples were collected from common room surfaces, personal items, and toilets, as well as high volume air samples and low volume personal air samples. Many commonly used items, toilet facilities, and air samples had evidence of viral contamination: 76.5% of all personal items and 80.4% of all room surfaces were positive for SARS-CoV-2 by RT-PCR (0.22-0.82 gene copies/microliter of swab resuspension); 63% of room air samples were positive (mean 2.86 copies/L of air); 81% of toilet samples were positive. The percentage of positive samples from each room ranged from 50% to 100%. There was no clear correlation between severity of illness, cough or fever, and the prevalence of viral RNA. Of note, air collectors positioned more than 6 feet from each of two patients yielded positive samples, as did air samplers placed outside patient rooms in the hallways. Although the results are preliminary, it appears that some samples are positive for infectious virus, including an air sample collected well more than 6 feet from a patient.[11] These results require urgent confirmation under a variety of conditions as they have significant implications for current public health messaging regarding necessary distancing between nearby individuals to prevent virus transmission. In addition, and in this case anecdotal, the highest airborne RNA concentrations were recorded by personal samplers while a patient was receiving oxygen through a nasal cannula (19.17 and 48.21 copies/L). The possibility of aerosol generation by oxygen delivery via nasal cannula and other mechanisms is currently being explored. Overall, these data support the possibilities of both direct (droplet and person-to-person) and indirect (contaminated objects, airborne) forms of transmission.

A recent study by Liu et al. provides additional information regarding aerodynamics, concentrations, and distribution of aerosols containing SARS-CoV-2.[12] A total of 35 aerosol samples (30 samples with total suspended particles, 3 samples with size-segregated particles, and 2 aerosol deposition samples) were collected in two hospitals and public areas in Wuhan, including patient areas, ICUs, medical staff areas, and toilet areas. In regard to patient areas, the highest concentrations of airborne SARS-CoV-2 were observed inside the patient mobile toilet room (19 copies m^{-3}), suggesting the importance of frequent disinfection of patient toilets. In regard to medical staff areas, the protective apparel removal rooms had the highest airborne virus concentrations (18 to 42 copies m^{-3}). In regard to public areas, airborne concentrations were generally below 3 copies m^{-3}, except for a crowded site near the entrance to a department store and a busy site next to a hospital. The peak concentrations of SARS-CoV-2 aerosols appear to exist in two distinct size ranges: 0.25 to 1.0 µm and those larger than 2.5 µm. Aerosols smaller than 2.5 µm can remain suspended in the air for many hours. The study observed that the negative pressure ventilation and high air exchange rate inside some locations were effective in minimizing airborne SARS-CoV-2. Additional findings suggest that virus-laden aerosol deposition may play a role in surface contamination and thus subsequent human infection. The authors believe that a direct source of SARS-CoV-2 may be due

---

[10] Santarpia et al. In preparation. Transmission potential of SARS-CoV-2 in viral shedding observed at the University of Nebraska Medical Center. Soon at *medRxiv*.

[11] Personal communication, Josh Santarpia, University of Nebraska Medical Center, March 25, 2020.

[12] Liu et al. 2020. Aerodynamic characteristics and RNA concentration of SARS-CoV-2 aerosol in Wuhan hospitals during COVID-19 outbreak. https://www.biorxiv.org/content/10.1101/2020.03.08.982637v1 (accessed March 26, 2020).

to a resuspension of virus-laden aerosol from the surface of medical staff protective apparel during removal, which may come from direct deposition of respiratory droplets while medical staff are working. Floor dust aerosol containing the virus is also subject to resuspension—meaning that virus-laden aerosols could first deposit on the surface of protective gear and then fall to the floor to be resuspended by medical staff movement. Outside of the hospital, only 2 crowd gathering sites (of 11 sites sampled) had detectable concentrations of SARS-CoV-2 aerosol, which may contribute to sources of virus-laden aerosol during sampling. It is important to note that the sample size for the aerosol samples, and notably the size-segregated samples (3) and aerosol deposition samples (2), were small—a limitation of this study. Furthermore, TRIzol LS Reagent (Invitrogen) was added to inactivate SARS-CoV-2 to extract the RNA, which should be noted as a limitation to the study because the authors measured viral RNA, not infectious virus.

There are a number of published studies that examine the relationship between the geographic incidence of COVID-19 cases and ambient temperature and humidity. Some suggest possible but modest correlations between geographies with higher temperature or humidity, and lower rates of disease; however, there are a number of confounding factors, including disease reporting practices and quality of and access to health care. We did not scrutinize these studies carefully nor perform an extensive search for related studies.

C. Caveats, Needs

A notable limitation of most of the natural history studies described above is a reliance on RT-PCR to assess the presence of SARS-CoV-2 on surfaces and air. Although viral RNA was detected in many environmental samples across the various studies, infectivity is not known. It is important to note that there are no available data to our knowledge that speak to the possible linkage between the presence of environmental viral RNA or even infectious virus and the risk of transmission from these environmental sites to humans. This is a key issue, and relates in part to another major issue and unanswered question: What is the infectious dose of SARS-CoV-2 for humans? Studies to address this question are planned, and in fact may be under way with non-human primates at several laboratories, but these studies will be limited by the relevance of non-human primate susceptibility to human susceptibility. The use of other laboratory animals will provide even less relevant information on incubation time.

Questions have been (appropriately) raised about whether there are relatively easy-to-perform, quick, and safe measurements one might undertake on environmental samples for predicting the presence of viable virus, rather than reliance on cultivation (PFU) assays. One idea recently discussed by Wölfel et al.[13] is to look for subgenomic mRNAs made by the virus during its life cycle in a human cell but not packaged into mature virions. These subgenomic mRNAs, if detected directly in a clinical sample, signify that the virus has been actively replicating in host cells in the sample at the time the sample was expelled from the body. This approach was used by Wölfel et al. to argue for active SARS-CoV-2 replication in the throat of COVID-19 patients during

---

[13] Wölfel et al. 2020. Virological assessment of hospitalized cases of coronavirus disease 2019. https://www.medrxiv.org/content/10.1101/2020.03.05.20030502v1.full.pdf (accessed March 25, 2020).

the first 5 days after symptoms onset. This approach could conceivably be used to assess the possibility of recent active viral replication in environmental swab samples.

An important caveat regarding the results from experimental studies relates to their relevance to real-world conditions. For example, many of the experimental environmental survival studies have used virus grown in TC media. It is quite possible that virus from naturally infected humans when directly disseminated to the nearby environment has different survival properties than virus grown in TC media, even when the latter is purified and spiked into a relevant human body fluid such as saliva. However, environmental dissemination of clinically relevant human fluids spiked with TC-grown virus will be more predictive of real-world environmental survival than environmental dissemination of TC-grown virus in TC media. Important human clinical matrices into which virus should be spiked include saliva, respiratory (including nasal) mucus and lower respiratory tract airway secretions, urine, blood, and stool. In addition, nebulized saline should be spiked and studied. Another issue related to experimental conditions is the effect of humidity on viral stability. Aerosol studies to date have tended to use humidity levels for culture media that are more favorable for viral decay (e.g., 50-65% relative humidity). Real respiratory fluid is likely to be more protective of infectivity, and indoor relative humidity in wintertime in temperate regions is usually 20-40%, a range that is more favorable for virus survival. Consequently, the half-lives reported to date may represent the lower end of the range. Differences in experimental conditions across studies (e.g., viral growth media, viral titer determination methods, infectivity of the inoculum) would be expected to contribute to variation in study results.

Before too many public health decisions are made on the basis of experimental or natural history studies using just one virus strain, some attention should be paid to the possibility of variation among different SARS-CoV-2 strains in their environmental survival properties. Different isolates from early and late in the pandemic, and from different geographic regions, should be studied and compared.

Registries of patient data and patient samples (e.g., nasopharyngeal, sera, urine, stool) are being created and can be used in future studies examining environmental persistence of the virus. For example, such samples could be used as clinical matrices to look at SARS-CoV-2 persistence on surfaces.

QUESTION 2: INCUBATION PERIOD

We approach this question in a similar way, examining first experimental studies and then natural history studies: (A) experimental studies, typically involving the inoculation of animals in the laboratory using a laboratory-propagated virus under controlled conditions and subsequent monitoring for onset of viral shedding, signs of disease, or other physiological responses; and (B) natural history studies, typically involving longitudinal or cross-sectional studies of naturally exposed humans and the collection of data on time of exposure and time of onset of signs, symptoms, and virological and molecular features of infection and disease. Each approach has strengths and weaknesses: with experimental studies there is control over time of exposure and various features of the inoculum, but non-human animals to varying degrees fail to reflect the natural history of infection in humans; with natural history studies, the host is relevant, but the time and nature of the exposure is less well understood and sample availability is uncertain.

A. Experimental Studies

As mentioned above, experimental infections in non-human primates are planned or are under way at several sites in the United States, including the Tulane University National Primate Research Center and RML,[14] and presumably in other countries. While animal models are very important for understanding pathogenesis and responses to therapeutic and vaccine candidates, they are not as helpful with the incubation period studies given physiological differences across species.

B. Natural History Studies

In a recent preprint from Shaanxi, China, and New York, Men et al. examined confirmed cases of COVID-19 from 10 regions in China, other than Hubei province, for whom there were data on time of exposure and time of disease onset.[15] A Monte Carlo simulation was employed to estimate incubation period, along with additional statistical analysis to assess relationships between different age and gender groups. In this study, the mean and median incubation periods were estimated to be 5.84 and 5.0 days, respectively. Patients 40 years or older had a longer incubation period and larger variance than did patients younger than 40 years. There was no statistically significant difference in incubation period based on gender. These findings suggest that different periods of quarantine may be advisable based on age. However, these results need to be confirmed through additional studies and with further stratification of incubation period results by age group.

In a recent preprint from the National Institute of Allergy and Infectious Diseases, Peking University, and the Chinese Center for Disease Control and Prevention, Qin et al. identified asymptomatic individuals at their time of departure from Wuhan and followed them until symptoms arose.[16] This method was reported to offer enhanced accuracy by reducing recall bias and by utilizing forward time data. More than 1,000 cases were collected from publicly available data. They found that the estimated median incubation period was 8.13 days, the mean was 8.62 days, the 90th percentile was 14.65 days, and the 99th percentile 20.59 days. Compared to other studies, this incubation period is longer. They conclude that ~10% of patients with COVID-19 do not develop symptoms until 14 days after infection.

In a recent preprint from Guangzhou and Hong Kong, He et al. reported on temporal patterns of viral shedding in 94 laboratory-confirmed COVID-19 patients and modeled COVID-19 infectiousness from a separate sample of 77 infector-infectee

---

[14] Personal communication, Chad Roy, Tulane University National Primate Research Center, March 24, 2020.

[15] Men et al. 2020. Estimate the incubation period of coronavirus 2019 (COVID-19). https://www.medrxiv.org/content/10.1101/2020.02.24.20027474v1.full.pdf (accessed March 25, 2020).

[16] Qin et al. 2020. Estimation of incubation period distribution of COVID-19 using disease onset forward time: A novel cross-sectional and forward follow-up study. https://www.medrxiv.org/content/10.1101/2020.03.06.20032417v1.full.pdf (accessed March 25, 2020).

transmission pairs.[17] They observed the highest viral load in throat swabs at the time of symptom onset, and inferred that infectiousness peaked on or before symptom onset. They estimated that 44% of transmissions may occur before the first symptoms of the index case.

C. Caveats, Needs

Robust estimates of the distribution of the incubation period and the period of infectiousness for SARS-CoV-2 are critically important to inform public health messaging. Differences in incubation period findings among existing studies may relate to methodological differences, limited sample sizes, recall bias, or inadequate follow-up (potentially missing people who have longer incubation periods). Given the small number of human studies evaluating these disease characteristics for COVID-19, additional studies to confirm incubation period estimates and infectiousness prior to symptom onset are urgently needed. For public health management, it makes a great deal of difference whether 1% of patients will develop the disease after 14 days (if the mean incubation is approximately 5 days) or whether the fraction is 10% of patients (if the mean incubation period is approximately 8 days). Additional studies should examine variables that may have an impact on incubation period, which, besides age (see Men et al. above), may include inoculum size, immune competency of host, co-infecting agents, and underlying morbid conditions. Prospective longitudinal studies are most effective for addressing this issue. An obvious challenge is precise identification and timing of natural exposures. Additionally, as mentioned above, it is conceivable that the evolution of new SARS-CoV-2 strain variants will be accompanied by different properties, including incubation period. Prior to changing current public health guidance, it may be prudent to compare observed incubation periods among different SARS-CoV-2 strains. Future studies related to incubation period and viral loads in asymptomatic patients may help to inform pressing questions related to, for example, the role of super spreaders and children in transmission.

Respectfully,
David A. Relman, M.D.
Member
Standing Committee on Emerging Infectious Diseases and 21st Century Health Threats

---

[17] He et al. 2020. Temporal dynamics in viral shedding and transmissibility of COVID-19. https://www.medrxiv.org/content/10.1101/2020.03.15.20036707v2.full.pdf (accessed March 25, 2020).

Rapid Expert Consultation on Crisis Standards of Care for the COVID-19 Pandemic (March 28, 2020)

March 28, 2020

ADM Brett Giroir, M.D.
Assistant Secretary for Health
200 Independence Avenue, SW
Washington, DC 20201

Robert Kadlec, M.D.
Assistant Secretary for Preparedness and Response
200 Independence Avenue, SW
Washington, DC 20201

Dear ADM Giroir and Dr. Kadlec:

Attached please find a rapid expert consultation that was prepared by the co-conveners of the Crisis Standards of Care working group, John Hick and Dan Hanfling, with input from others listed in the attachment, and conducted under the auspices of the National Academies of Sciences, Engineering, and Medicine's Standing Committee on Emerging Infectious Diseases and 21st Century Health Threats.

Building on the previous decade of National Academies reports, the aim of this rapid expert consultation is to articulate the guiding principles, key elements, and core messages that undergird Crisis Standards of Care decision making at all levels. It does not, and in our opinion should not, attempt to dictate exactly what choice should be made under exactly what circumstance, as that depends on the specific circumstances of the case at hand, and these must be left to the judgment of the professional, institutional, community, and civic leaders who are best situated to understand the local reality.

In my opinion, one of the most important components of the rapid expert consultation is the core principle derived from earlier reports, namely, that Crisis Standards of Care compel thinking in terms of what is best for an entire group of patients, on the principle of saving the most lives (or achieving the best outcome for the group of patients) rather than focusing only on an individual patient under your care. When equipment, staffing, and material are sufficient, focusing only on what is best for each individual patient is tantamount to the best outcome for the collection of patients because the group outcome is simply the sum of the individual outcomes. Under conditions that compel Crisis Standards of Care, this identity of outcomes for the individual and group breaks down, and the decision makers cannot avoid the hard choices before them. We hope these principles, elements, and messages can assist in discussing and making these difficult, heart-rending decisions.

Respectfully,
Harvey V. Fineberg, M.D., Ph.D.
Chair
Standing Committee on Emerging Infectious Diseases and 21st Century Health Threats

This rapid expert consultation responds to your March 25 request to provide a rationale for the implementation of crisis standards of care (CSC) in response to the COVID-19 outbreak. Also discussed are the broad principles and core elements of CSC planning and implementation. This discussion builds on a 10-year foundation of three seminal reports on CSC issued in 2009, 2012, and 2013 by the Institute of Medicine (IOM), which are described in Appendix A at the end of this document.

This document is meant to provide principles and guidance. It is neither appropriate nor feasible for us to detail actual choices and preferences that apply to specific situations, each of which depends on the exigencies of the epidemic relative to locally available facilities, equipment, personnel, and other needed resources. Rather, this document describes the basis upon which to carry out such decision making whenever it has to happen.

Catastrophic emergencies are by their very nature disruptive and life altering. They can have far-reaching societal impacts, even challenging fundamental assumptions about how we live and what we take for granted. Nowhere is this more evident than when medical facilities cannot deliver the usual level of care to all those who need medical attention. This is the current and likely future reality for many institutions caring for the growing numbers of patients with SARS-CoV-2 infection.

CRISIS STANDARDS OF CARE DEFINITION, GUIDING PRINCIPLES, AND KEY ELEMENTS OF PLANNING

Crisis standards of care are applied when a pervasive or catastrophic disaster make it impossible to meet usual health care standards.

GUIDING PRINCIPLES

- Health care planning must do everything possible never to need CSC.
- CSC have the joint goals of extending the availability of key resources and minimizing the impact of shortages on clinical care.
- CSC strive to save the most lives possible, recognizing that some individual patients will die, who would survive under usual care.
- Implementation of CSC will require facility-specific decisions regarding the allocation of limited resources, including how patients will be triaged to receive life-saving care.

KEY ELEMENTS OF CSC PLANNING

Ethical Grounding

- During a catastrophic crisis, it is vitally important to uphold the core ethical principles of fairness, duty to care, duty to steward resources, transparency in decision making, consistency, proportionality, and accountability.
- When resource scarcity reaches catastrophic levels, clinicians are ethically justified—and, indeed, are ethically obligated—to use the available resources to sustain life and well-being to the greatest extent possible.

Engagement, Education, and Communication

- CSC planning must involve both providers and the public in order to ensure the legitimacy of the process and the standards.
- These CSC planning processes must be proactive, honest, transparent, and accountable regarding the state of the U.S. health care system as COVID-19 cases increase, in order to warrant the public's trust.
- Senior leadership must prepare health care workers for the possible need for CSC and support them as they face the decisions that violate usual care standards.

continued

Legal Considerations

- Health care workers who must make difficult decisions implementing CSC must have adequate guidance and legal protections.
- Under disaster conditions, adherence to core constitutional principles remains a constant, but other statutory or regulatory provisions can be altered as necessary in real time.

Indicators, Triggers, and Responsibility
(Examples of hospital indicators, triggers, and tactics for transitions along the continuum of care are outlined in Appendix A.)

- Institutions must be alert to indicators that signal a shift to CSC levels of care.
- Observation of those indicators should trigger plans for initiating the contingency or crisis care standards.

Evidence-Based Clinical Operations

- Decisions made at the bedside should be evidence-based.
- Current predictive scoring systems of patient outcomes have unclear value in the COVID-19 context.
- Evidence-based care guidelines may emerge over the course of the pandemic, and with them, CSC guidelines should also evolve, if feasible.

Shifting to CSC is the only ethically tenable approach to shortages of health care resources. Ultimately, this shift represents not a rejection of ethical principles but their embodiment.

THE CONTINUUM OF CARE

Standards of care fall along a continuum of three levels, reflecting the incremental surge in demand relative to available health care resources:

- *Conventional care* is everyday health care services.
- *Contingency care* arises when demand for medical staff, equipment, or pharmaceuticals begins to exceed supply. Contingency care seeks functionally equivalent care, recognizing that some adjustments to usual care are necessary.
- *Crisis care* occurs when resources are so depleted that functionally equivalent care is no longer possible.

Appendix A provides examples of the kinds of shortages that can trigger CSC.

THE GOAL OF CSC PLANNING

The transition from conventional to contingency to crisis care comes with a concomitant increase in morbidity and mortality. Thus, it is crucial that planning ensure that

CSC is never needed, proactively moving resources ahead of when they are needed. When the system is at risk of becoming overwhelmed, the goal then becomes to conserve, substitute, adapt, and reuse, so that, only in the most extreme of circumstances, are CSC needed.

THE KEY ELEMENTS OF CSC PLANNING

Here, we elaborate briefly on the five key elements of CSC planning:

- A strong ethical grounding;
- Integrated, continuing community and provider engagement, education, and communication;
- Assurances regarding legal authority and environment;
- Clear indicators, triggers, and lines of responsibility; and
- Evidence-based clinical processes and operations.

Ethical Grounding. During a crisis, it is vitally important to adhere to core ethical principles: fairness, the duty to care, the duty to steward resources, transparency in decision making, consistency, proportionality, and accountability. Medical decisions informed by these ethical principles may allow for actions that would be unacceptable under ordinary circumstances, such as not providing some patients with resources when other patients would derive greater benefit from them. When resource scarcity reaches catastrophic levels, clinicians are ethically justified—and indeed are ethically obligated—to use the available resources to sustain life and well-being to the greatest extent possible.

Engagement, Education, and Communication. Both providers and the public must be engaged in CSC planning both to ensure the legitimacy of the process and the resulting standards and to achieve the best possible result. Both the public and health care providers must understand these difficult choices and be engaged in developing the criteria for making them. Those criteria must then be clear enough that practitioners can apply them when making decisions at the bedside, especially when the stewarding of scarce resources means withholding or withdrawing critical care services. Those criteria must reflect the values, wishes, and interests of all patients, especially the most vulnerable.

In the current pandemic, public trust is essential. To this end, health care leaders must be proactive, honest, transparent, and accountable when communicating the state of their institutions and the system as a whole. Given the resources available at the start of the crisis and expected during the immediate period, demand for health care services, especially in critical care, will soon outstrip health care providers' ability to deliver usual care in many communities, as has already occurred in several metropolitan areas. Reports on extreme conditions elsewhere may not prepare the public for the shift to CSC in their own hometowns. Health care and political leaders have a duty to forewarn the public about what is coming, and the implications of CSC.

Senior leaders must also provide material and moral support to health care workers, who will bear the physical, health, and psychological burdens of working under CSC conditions. Providing that support will require careful, consistent messaging; ongoing two-way communication; and attention to the needs created by grueling, stressful work.

Legal Considerations. The law must inform CSC and create incentives for protecting the public's health and respecting individual rights. Extreme scarcity can necessitate difficult life-and-death decisions. Health care workers who will have to make them must have adequate guidance and legal protections. They must be able to follow the rule of law, even under disaster conditions.

At the same time, health care workers must be continually and clearly informed about all relevant changes in statutory or regulatory provisions. These legal issues may affect (1) the organization of key personnel, (2) fair access to treatment, (3) coordination of services within and across health systems, (4) assurance of patients' interests, (5) allocation of scarce resources, (6) protection of health care workers and volunteers from unwarranted liability claims, (7) reimbursement of costs incurred when protecting the public's health, and (8) interjurisdictional cooperation and coordination.

Indicators, Triggers, and Responsibility. Communities must be alert to indicators that signal a shift in the level of care that can be delivered. Under pandemic conditions, changes can occur rapidly. Being as prepared as possible requires situational awareness, open lines of practical and risk communication, and clear lines of authority and responsibility. Appendix A provides examples of such signals.

Evidence-Based Clinical Operations (Making Clinical Decisions Under Crisis Conditions). Bedside decisions should be evidence-based, drawing on clinical research and experience as consistently and transparently as possible. These should evolve as evidence accrues. For the current situation, existing prospective tools are insufficient for decision making. For example, Sequential Organ Failure Assessment (SOFA) scores have proven to be poor predictors of individual patients' survival, particularly for those with primary respiratory failure. Hence, at their current state of development, these scores are not suitable for excluding patients with respiratory failure from SARS-CoV-2 from receiving critical care. Similar reservations apply to other currently available decision support tools, although their value may improve as experience accumulates with patients having SARS-CoV-2 infection. Even in the face of imperfect data, decision making will be needed at multiple levels. Governments and institutions should consider these criteria proactively, and disseminate them publicly and transparently. This will permit public input and enable better response to evolving science and local circumstances. A useful summary of ethical guidelines and list of resources has been compiled by The Hastings Center.[1]

It is important to separate triage at each level of care from care provided at the bedside. This enables caregivers to better fulfill their ethical obligations to individual patients, while other decision-making processes ensure care provides the greatest good for the greatest number. Governments at all levels, institutions, and frontline caregivers

---

[1] Berlinger et al. 2020. Ethical framework for health care institutions & guidelines for institutional ethics services responding to the coronavirus pandemic: Managing uncertainty, safeguarding communities, guiding practice. The Hastings Center. https://www.thehastingscenter.org/ethicalframeworkcovid19.

should recognize that these decisions are difficult and inherently involve ethical concerns. Ongoing peer and psychological support for those involved will be essential for them to continue their work.

THE BOTTOM LINE

Despite efforts to forestall the spread of SARS-CoV-2 to date, it appears that the COVID-19 outbreak will continue expanding across the United States. We can, therefore, anticipate that a growing number of hospitals will face medical needs that outpace the existing supply of ventilators, protective equipment, and other essentials, as well as the rate that enhanced supply can be produced, acquired, and put into place. These circumstances will require a shift to CSC.

Preparing for CSC means taking all feasible measures—including reuse, substitution, conservation, and administrative controls—to prevent or delay the need for CSC as long as possible. These measures must be taken at all levels of government, the health care system, and society. There is also an imminent need to prepare for difficult decisions about allocating limited resources, triaging patients to receive life-saving care, and minimizing the negative impacts of delivering care under crisis conditions. These preparations and the decisions that arise from them should be transparent and shared with the public. We hope the principles and elements of CSC planning outlined here will help decision makers at all levels.

Preparations for CSC include trustworthy communication with all stakeholders. Both the content and the process of those communications must convey the messages in the box below, which summarize the principles in the three seminal IOM reports on CSC. Failure to communicate regarding the shift to CSC will diminish public trust in health care providers and systems, as well as in government leadership. Without clear, consistent, candid communication, lost faith in institutions could become one more victim of COVID-19.

KEY MESSAGES AND PRINCIPLES

The following key messages and principles drawn from the three seminal Institute of Medicine (IOM) reports, described in Appendix A, can serve as a starting point for introducing the commitments of those responsible for the shift to CSC in response to COVID-19:

- **We, the health care community, are doing everything possible to prevent and avoid crisis conditions and maintain conventional standards of care.** We are partners with the rest of society in slowing the spread of disease to decrease the number of people who may need critical care at the same time.

continued

- **We recognize that the principal goal of implementing CSC is to maximize benefits to society, which includes saving as many lives—patients, health care workers, and front-line first responders—as possible.** CSC decisions allocate scarce treatment resources to those patients who are most likely to benefit, consistent with community values as articulated by bodies convened for this purpose (see Appendix A). Applying this overarching principle requires wise stewardship of medical resources, so that health care workers can help as many patients as possible. They need government, business, and health care systems to increase the supply and timely delivery of needed resources.
- **We are committed to creating CSC strategies that are fair, equitable, and responsive in order to maximize the safety of providers and patients.** Fairness is of paramount importance in the allocation of scarce life-saving medical resources.
- **We will communicate CSC in clear, consistent terms, through channels relevant to diverse stakeholder audiences.** We will speak with one voice to convey governmental commitment to a deliberate, thoughtful process on making these decisions of grave importance. We will draw on relevant research and community experience.
- **We anticipate that conditions will change as the pandemic spreads nationally, leading to dynamic shifts in standards of care, across communities and facilities.** We will apply the best available science to forecast those needs, address them equitably, and communicate the rationale for our actions.
- **We will consider patient and family preferences insofar as possible, within the constraint of allocating resources with the goal of saving the most patient and provider lives.** We will respect patients' dignity and preserve their comfort in all instances.
- **We will prepare adequately for the emotional impacts of CSC on health care workers, patients, their loved ones, and the public as a whole.** We will address the behavioral health needs of health care workers, patients, and their families, knowing the distress that CSC decisions will bring. We will explain these decisions and demonstrate empathy with the distress and losses.

Respectfully,
John Hick, M.D.
Member
Standing Committee on Emerging Infectious Diseases and 21st Century Health Threats

Dan Hanfling, M.D.
Co-Chair
2009, 2012, and 2013 Institute of Medicine Crisis Standards of Care committees

APPENDIX A

Foundational Work of the Institute of Medicine

A decade ago, during the period between the first and second waves of the H1N1 pandemic, the Institute of Medicine (IOM) convened a committee to address the following fundamental questions related to crisis standards of care (CSC):

- Who should receive care when not all who need it can be attended to?
- How should decisions be made about who gets access to care?
- Should the standard of care change to reflect the care that can be delivered under such circumstances?

The answers to these core questions formed the basis for the recommendations in the IOM's 2009 Letter Report.[2] One of those recommendations was to "enable specific legal/regulatory powers and protections for health care providers in the necessary tasks of allocating and using scarce medical resources and implementing alternate care facilities" in the response to such events. The Letter Report also emphasized that CSC should be "formally declared by a state government" in recognition that crisis care operations "will be in place for a sustained period of time."

Building on this work, the IOM in 2012 issued a report[3] articulating a systems framework for catastrophic disaster planning and response, highlighting specific steps that key stakeholders—hospitals and health systems, public health and public safety agencies, emergency medical services, and providers of outpatient medical services—would need to take to prepare for health care delivery under crisis conditions. The third report, published in 2013,[4] focused on the development of a toolkit identifying the indicators, triggers, and tactics needed to transition from conventional care to CSC.

These reports are as timely and relevant today as they were the day they were released. The conditions under which CSC must be considered as a possibility clearly exist today, given the rapid spread of COVID-19 in communities across the United States and the resulting declarations of a public health emergency by U.S. Department of Health and Human Services Secretary Azar; a national emergency by President Trump; and emergency declarations by every U.S. state and territory, as well as hundreds of municipalities.[5]

All decision makers engaged in the response to the COVID-19 outbreak will be challenged to answer crucial, complex questions reflecting the ethical, legal, clinical, political, and societal dimensions of this crisis. They will need to make difficult decisions about the allocation of resources, decisions with life-and-death consequences. The

---

[2] Institute of Medicine. 2009. *Guidance for Establishing Crisis Standards of Care for Use in Disaster Situations: A Letter Report*. Washington, DC: The National Academies Press. https://doi.org/10.17226/12749.

[3] Institute of Medicine. 2012. *Crisis Standards of Care: A Systems Framework for Catastrophic Disaster Response: Volume 1: Introduction and CSC Framework*. Washington, DC: The National Academies Press. https://doi.org/10.17226/13351.

[4] Institute of Medicine. 2013. *Crisis Standards of Care: A Toolkit for Indicators and Triggers*. Washington, DC: The National Academies Press. https://doi.org/10.17226/18338.

[5] Descriptions of the emergency, disaster, and public health emergency categories can be found at https://www.networkforphl.org/resources/emergency-legal-preparedness-covid19.

CSC framework, expressed in the recommendations and guidance of the IOM reports constitute the foundation for this rapid expert consultation and can guide our nation's response.

APPENDIX B

Authors and Reviewers of This Rapid Expert Consultation

This rapid expert consultation was prepared by Dan Hanfling, In-Q-Tel, and John Hick, Hennepin County Medical Center, as the co-conveners of the CSC working group under the auspices of the National Academies' Standing Committee on Emerging Infectious Diseases and 21st Century Health Threats. The working group for this document included the following individuals: Donald Berwick, Institute for Healthcare Improvement; Richard Besser, Robert Wood Johnson Foundation; Carlos del Rio, Emory Vaccine Center; James Hodge, Arizona State University; Kent Kester, Sanofi Pasteur; Jennifer Nuzzo, Johns Hopkins Bloomberg School of Public Health; Tara O'Toole, In-Q-Tel; Richard Serino, Harvard T.H. Chan School of Public Health; Beth Weaver, RESOLVE; and Matthew Wynia, University of Colorado Center for Bioethics and Humanities.

Harvey Fineberg, chair of the Standing Committee, approved this document. The following individuals served as reviewers: Baruch Fischhoff, Carnegie Mellon University; Bernard Lo, The Greenwall Foundation; Nicole Lurie, Coalition for Epidemic Preparedness Innovations and Harvard University; and Monica Schoch-Spana, Johns Hopkins Bloomberg School of Public Health. Ellen Wright Clayton, Vanderbilt University Medical University, and Susan Curry, University of Iowa, served as arbiters of this review on behalf of the National Academies' Report Review Committee and their Health and Medicine Division.

Rapid Expert Consultation on the Possibility of Bioaerosol Spread of SARS-CoV-2 for the COVID-19 Pandemic (April 1, 2020)

April 1, 2020

Kelvin Droegemeier, Ph.D.
Office of Science and Technology Policy
Executive Office of the President
Eisenhower Executive Office Building
1650 Pennsylvania Avenue, NW
Washington, DC 20504

Dear Dr. Droegemeier:

This letter responds to your question concerning the possibility that SARS-CoV-2 could be spread by conversation, in addition to sneeze/cough-induced droplets.

Currently available research supports the possibility that SARS-CoV-2 could be spread via bioaerosols generated directly by patients' exhalation. One must be cautious in imputing the findings with one respiratory virus to another respiratory virus, as each virus may have its own effective infectious inoculum and distinct aerosolization characteristics. Studies that rely on polymerase chain reaction (PCR) to detect the presence of viral RNA may not represent viable virus in sufficient amounts to produce infection. Nevertheless, the presence of viral RNA in air droplets and aerosols indicates the possibility of viral transmission via these routes.

A recent study of SARS-CoV-2 aerosolization at the University of Nebraska Medical Center showed widespread presence of viral RNA in isolation rooms where patients with SARS-CoV-2 were receiving care. Santarpia et al. collected air and surface samples from 11 isolation rooms that were used to care for patients infected with SARS-CoV-2. Included in that study were both high volume air samples and low volume personal air samples. Of note, air collectors positioned more than 6 feet from each of two patients yielded samples positive for viral RNA when evaluated using reverse-transcriptase PCR (RT-PCR), as did air samplers placed outside patient rooms in the hallways. Personal collectors worn by samplers also were positive even though patients were not coughing while samplers were present. Anecdotally, the highest airborne RNA concentrations were recorded by personal samplers while a patient was receiving oxygen through a nasal cannula (19.17 and 48.21 copies/L). While this research indicates that viral particles can be spread via bioaerosols, the authors stated that finding infectious virus has proved elusive and experiments are ongoing to determine viral activity in the collected samples.[1]

An airflow modeling study following the SARS-CoV-1 outbreak in Hong Kong in the early 2000s supports the potential for transmission via bioaerosols. In that study, the significantly increased risk of infection to residents on higher floors of a building that was home to an infected individual indicated to the researchers a pattern of infection consistent with a rising plume of contaminated warm air.[2]

In a recent study conducted at the University of Hong Kong, not yet subject to peer review, Leung et al collected respiratory droplets and aerosols from children and adults with acute respiratory illnesses with and without surgical masks. The investigators found human coronaviruses [other than SARS-CoV-2], influenza virus, and rhinovirus from both aerosols and respiratory droplets. Surgical masks reduced detection of coronavirus RNA in both respiratory droplets and aerosols, but only respiratory droplets and not aerosols for influenza virus RNA. These findings suggest that surgical face masks could reduce the transmission of human coronavirus and influenza infections if worn by infected individuals capable of transmitting the infection.[3]

A study of SARS-CoV-2 raises concerns about transmission via aerosols generated from droplet contaminated surfaces. Liu et al. collected 35 aerosol samples in 2 hospitals and public areas in Wuhan. From samples collected in patient care areas the highest concentration of the virus was found in toilet facilities (19 copies m^{-3}), and in medical staff areas the highest concentrations were identified in personal protective equipment (PPE) removal rooms (18-42 copies m^{-3}). By comparison, in all but two crowded sites, the concentrations of the virus found in public areas was below 3 copies m^{-3}. The authors conclude that a direct source of SARS-CoV-2 may be a virus-laden aerosol resuspended by the doffing of PPE, the cleaning of floors, or the movement of staff.[4] It may be difficult to resuspend particles of a respirable size. However, fomites could be transmitted to the hands, mouth, nose, or eyes without requiring direct respiration into the lungs.

---

[1] Santarpia et al. 2020. Transmission potential of SARS-CoV-2 in viral shedding observed at the University of Nebraska Medical Center. https://www.medrxiv.org/content/10.1101/2020.03.23.20039446v2.

[2] Yu et al. 2004. Evidence of airborne transmission of the severe acute respiratory syndrome virus. *New England Journal of Medicine* 350:1731-1739. DOI: 10.1056/NEJMoa032867.

[3] Leung et al. 2020. Respiratory virus shedding in exhaled breath and efficacy of face masks. Under review. DOI: 10.21203/rs.3.rs-16836/v1.

[4] Liu et al. 2020. Aerodynamic characteristics and RNA concentration of SARS-CoV-2 aerosol in Wuhan hospitals during COVID-19 outbreak. https://www.biorxiv.org/content/10.1101/2020.03.08.982637v1.

Individuals vary in the degree to which they produce bioaerosols through normal breathing.[5] This may have a bearing on efficiency of transmission of SARS-CoV-2 by different infected but asymptomatic individuals.

Additional research specific to the aerosolization of SARS-CoV-2 during breathing and speech, the behavior of SARS-CoV-2 containing aerosols in the environment, both from laboratory studies and clinical experience, and the infectivity of bioaerosols containing SARS-CoV-2, would provide a more complete understanding of the level of risk of transmission of SARS-CoV-2 via bioaerosols spread by exhalation and normal speech. However, for no respiratory virus is the exact proportion of infections due to air droplet, aerosol, or fomite transmission fully established, and many individual factors and situations may contribute to the importance of each route of transmission.

While the current SARS-CoV-2 specific research is limited, the results of available studies are consistent with aerosolization of virus from normal breathing.

This response was prepared by staff of the National Academies of Sciences, Engineering, and Medicine based on a rapid review of the available literature and input from me. Georges Benjamin, American Public Health Association, and Ed Nardell, Harvard University, contributed to this response. Bobbie Berkowitz, Columbia University School of Nursing, and Ellen Wright Clayton, Vanderbilt University Medical University, reviewed and approved this document on behalf of the National Academies' Report Review Committee and their Health and Medicine Division.

My colleagues and I hope this input is helpful to you as you continue to guide the nation's response in this ongoing public health crisis.

Respectfully,
Harvey V. Fineberg, M.D., Ph.D.
Chair
Standing Committee on Emerging Infectious Diseases and 21st Century Health Threats

---

[5] Edwards et al. 2004. Inhaling to mitigate exhaled bioaerosols. *PNAS* 101(50):17383-17388. DOI: 10.1073/pnas.0408159101.

Rapid Expert Consultation on SARS-CoV-2 Survival in Relation to Temperature and Humidity and Potential for Seasonality for the COVID-19 Pandemic (April 7, 2020)

April 7, 2020

Kelvin Droegemeier, Ph.D.
Office of Science and Technology Policy
Executive Office of the President
Eisenhower Executive Office Building
1650 Pennsylvania Avenue, NW
Washington, DC 20504

Dear Dr. Droegemeier:

Attached please find a rapid expert consultation on the topics of virus survival in relation to temperature and humidity and potential for seasonal reduction and resurgence of cases. This assessment was prepared by members of the National Academies of Sciences, Engineering, and Medicine's Standing Committee on Emerging Infectious Diseases and 21st Century Health Threats.

The aim of this rapid expert consultation is to provide scientifically grounded principles that are relevant to decision making about the potential for seasonal variation of SARS-CoV-2.

We hope this document proves useful to you and your colleagues.

Respectfully,
Harvey V. Fineberg, M.D., Ph.D.
Chair
Standing Committee on Emerging Infectious Diseases and 21st Century Health Threats

This rapid expert consultation responds to your request concerning (1) survival of SARS-CoV-2 in relation to temperature and humidity; and (2) potential for seasonal reduction and resurgence in cases.[1]

In general, a common approach to issue 1 is with experimental studies in the laboratory, typically involving the deliberate dissemination of a laboratory-propagated virus under controlled environmental conditions with subsequent sampling. The most common approach to issue 2 is with natural history studies that observe disease transmission in different locations and times of year and seek correlations with environmental conditions such as temperature and humidity. Each approach has strengths and weaknesses: with experimental studies, environmental conditions can be controlled, but almost always the conditions fail to adequately mimic those of the natural setting; with natural history studies, the conditions are relevant and reflect the real world, but there is typically little control of environmental conditions and there are many confounding factors. Because the two approaches are so distinct, it is often difficult to harmonize the findings from the two, and relate the findings from one to the other.

LABORATORY STUDIES

In the *Rapid Expert Consultation Update on SARS-CoV-2 Surface Stability and Incubation for the COVID-19 Pandemic (March 27, 2020)* we reviewed laboratory studies of SARS-CoV-2 survival under controlled environmental conditions. We provide a slightly updated version of that review here. We note that since the March 27 rapid expert consultation, there is minimal new information published on this topic (e.g., one preprint is now published). Work is ongoing, but no results have been made available.

The laboratory data available so far indicate reduced survival of SARS-CoV-2 at elevated temperatures and variation in temperature sensitivity as a function of the type of surface on which the virus is placed. However, the number of well-controlled studies on the topic available at this time remains small. We anticipate new, relevant data within the next week or two, and in particular, data on surface survival of the virus under different levels of humidity, and aerosol survival with and without exposure to natural levels of ultraviolet (UV) radiation.

In a now published report from Hong Kong, Chin et al. examined the stability (using viral culture) of SARS-CoV-2 as a function of temperature, type of surface, and following the use of disinfectants.[2] With respect to temperature, using a starting suspension of 6.7 log $TCID_{50}$/ml in virus transport medium,[3] at 4°C there was only a 0.6-log unit reduction at the end of 14 days of incubation in this medium; at 22°C, a 3-log unit reduction after 7 days, and no detection at 14 days; and at 37°C, a 3-log unit reduction after 1 day and no virus detected afterward. No virus was detected after 30 minutes at 56°C or after 5 minutes at 70°C. With respect to survival on surfaces using a 5 µL droplet of virus culture at 7.8 log $TCID_{50}$/ml, no infectious virus was recovered from printing and tissue paper after 3 hours; no infectious virus was detected on cloth after

---

[1] A previous iteration of this rapid expert consultation is available upon request from SCEID@nas.edu. The previous iteration did not include the discussion on laboratory studies.

[2] Chin et al. Stability of SARS-CoV-2 in different environmental conditions. Lancet Microbe 2020. https://doi.org/10.1016/S2666-5247(20)30003-3.

[3] $TCID_{50}$ is the Median Tissue Culture Infectious Dose.

2 days or on stainless steel after 7 days. However, on the outside of a surgical mask, 0.1% of the original inoculum was detected on day 7. The persistence of infectious virus on personal protective equipment (PPE) is concerning and warrants additional study to inform guidance for health care workers. Such studies should also examine the effects of various treatments that might be used to disinfect PPE when they cannot be discarded after single use.

Chad Roy from the Tulane University National Primate Research Center shared via telephone some preliminary results of dynamic aerosol stability experiments with SARS-CoV-2 conducted over the past several weeks at the Infectious Disease Aerobiology Core program at Tulane.[4] His group generated an aerosol with a fairly uniform distribution of 2 micron particles, using virus grown in DMEM tissue culture (TC) medium and suspended in a rotating drum at an ambient temperature of ~23ºC and ~50% humidity. The aerosol was sampled longitudinally for up to 16 hours, and the virus was assessed for viability by growth (enumeration of plaque forming units [PFUs]) and morphology (electron microscopy). He reports surprisingly that SARS-CoV-2 has a longer half-life under these conditions than influenza virus, SARS-CoV-1, monkeypox virus, and *Mycobacterium tuberculosis*. As of March 24, he was waiting for some growth results, but expected to post a manuscript describing these findings to bioRxiv soon. This result is also concerning, but is quite preliminary; importantly, the details have not yet been shared.

George Korch and Mike Hevey from the National Biodefense Analysis and Countermeasures Center (NBACC), which was created by the U.S. Department of Homeland Security, shared their plans for an extensive series of experiments on SARS-CoV-2 environmental survival.[5] Because they share their plans with the White House Coronavirus Task Force, only a few observations are provided here. The NBACC is well suited for the kinds of studies it has planned, and the scope and relevance are noteworthy. In particular, it plans to create simulated infected body fluids, including saliva and lower respiratory secretions. It plans to test simulated solar radiation on virus survival, which is important. It also has already examined a wider range of relative humidity and temperature than some other groups, which is again, important. And it will compare RNA semi-quantitative measurements with viral growth (PFUs) on samples from all conditions, which is critical.

At Rocky Mountain Laboratories (RML), part of the National Institutes of Health, current studies include the effect of temperature and humidity on virus stability; virus stability in human body fluids, including urine and feces; and the effectiveness of decontamination procedures for PPE, including N95 respirators.[6]

There are important caveats regarding the results from experimental studies. The first caveat concerns the relevance of laboratory conditions to real-world conditions. For example, many of the experimental survival studies have used virus grown in TC media. One expects that virus from naturally infected humans when directly disseminated to the nearby environment has different survival properties than virus grown

---

[4] Personal communication, Chad Roy, Tulane University National Primate Research Center, March 24, 2020.

[5] Personal communication, George Korch and Mike Hevey, National Biodefense Analysis and Countermeasures Center, March 24, 2020.

[6] Personal communication, Vincent Munster, Rocky Mountain Laboratories, March 24, 2020.

in TC media, even when the latter is purified and spiked into a relevant human body fluid such as saliva. Having said this, environmental dissemination of clinically relevant human fluids spiked with TC-grown virus will be more predictive of real-world virus survival than environmental dissemination of TC-grown virus in TC media. Important human clinical matrices into which virus should be spiked include saliva, respiratory (including nasal) mucus and lower respiratory tract airway secretions, urine, blood, and stool. In addition, nebulized saline should be spiked and studied.

Another issue is humidity and the failure or inability of some laboratories to control and vary relative humidity for their experiments. For example, the Tulane Infectious Disease Aerobiology Core lab cannot vary humidity in a controlled fashion; whereas the NBACC is able to do so. Aerosol studies to date have typically used TC-grown virus and have therefore used humidity levels that are more favorable for viral decay (e.g., 50-65% relative humidity). Real respiratory fluid is likely to be more protective of infectivity, and indoor relative humidity in wintertime in temperate regions is usually 20-40%, a range that is more favorable for virus survival. Consequently, the half-lives reported to date under these conditions may represent the lower end of the range. Differences in experimental conditions across studies (e.g., viral growth media, viral titer determination methods, infectivity of the inoculum) would be expected to contribute to variation in study results.

Finally, attention should be paid to the possibility of variation in environmental survival among different SARS-CoV-2 strains. Isolates from early and late in the pandemic and from different geographic regions should be studied and compared.

NATURAL HISTORY STUDIES

Studies published so far have conflicting results regarding potential seasonal effects and are hampered by poor data quality, confounding factors, and insufficient time since the beginning of the pandemic from which to draw conclusions. There is some evidence to suggest that SARS-CoV-2 may transmit less efficiently in environments with higher ambient temperature and humidity; however, given the lack of host immunity globally, this reduction in transmission efficiency may not lead to a significant reduction in disease spread without the concomitant adoption of major public health interventions. Furthermore, the other coronaviruses causing potentially serious human illness, including both SARS-CoV and MERS-CoV, have not demonstrated any evidence of seasonality following their emergence.

The current pandemic started in the winter season mostly in northern latitudes, and less than 4 months ago, making it difficult to ascertain differences within a localized geographic region with changing seasons. Some analyses of variability across different geographic regions based on humidity and temperature are available. A study from China in the early part of the pandemic suggested that every 1°C elevation in ambient temperature led to a decrease in daily confirmed cases by 36-57% when relative humidity was between 67% to 85.5%, and every 1% increase in relative humidity decreased the daily confirmed cases by 11-22% when the average temperature was between 5.04°C and 8.2°C, but these findings were not consistent across mainland

China.[7] Another study in China concluded that increases in temperature and relative humidity can lower the reproductive rate, but the average R_0 was still close to 2 at maximum temperatures and humidity in their dataset, suggesting that the virus will still spread exponentially at higher temperatures and humidity.[8] Outside of China, a study looking at daily case growth rates in 121 countries or regions found the highest rates in temperate regions.[9] They found growth rates peaked in regions with a mean temperature of 5°C and decreased in warmer and colder climates. Temperature was the variable with the highest relative importance in explaining variations in growth rates although they did see fast growth rates in warmer climates and huge variations in regions with similar climates, suggesting that many factors contribute to transmission. Another study in 310 geographic regions across 116 countries also found an inverse relationship between temperature and humidity and incidence of COVID-19.[10] One study examined cities with significant community spread compared to those without spread and found greater disease rates in cities and regions along a narrow distribution within the 30-50° N' corridor (areas of lower average temperature and humidity), which is consistent with the behavior of seasonal respiratory viruses.[11] A study in countries that had at least 12 days of data found an increase in doubling time of virus transmission at warmer temperatures (average of 9.5°C versus 26.5°C), suggesting a slowing of disease spread at warmer temperatures.[12]

The results of these studies should be interpreted with caution, in the context of the limited time during which natural experiments have taken place in different locations. There are significant caveats in all of the studies presented, mostly related to data quality and the limitation in time and location, with the pandemic mostly in temperate regions during the winter months. Issues with data quality include the estimates of reproductive rate, assumptions about infectivity period, and short observational time windows. There are also important confounding factors associated with geography and hence, with temperature and humidity: access to and quality of public health and health care systems, per capita income, human behavioral patterns, and the availability of diagnostics. As a reflection of these confounding factors, those studies that show a significant correlation between temperature and humidity and disease transmission, also show that the two factors explain only a small fraction of the overall variation in transmission rates. Of note, a study by Luo et al. showed sustained transmission despite changes in weather in various parts of China that ranged from cold and dry to tropical arguing against any seasonal differences, although issues with data collection and

---

[7] Qi et al. 2020. COVID-19 transmission in Mainland China is associated with temperature and humidity: A time-series analysis. https://doi.org/10.1101/2020.03.30.20044099.

[8] Wang et al. 2020. High temperature and high humidity reduce the transmission of COVID-19. http://dx.doi.org/10.2139/ssrn.3551767.

[9] Ficetola and Rubolini. 2020. Climate affects global patterns of COVID-19 early outbreak dynamics. https://doi.org/10.1101/2020.03.23.20040501.

[10] Islam et al. 2020. Temperature, humidity, and wind speed are associated with lower COVID-19 incidence. https://doi.org/10.1101/2020.03.27.20045658.

[11] Sajadi et al. 2020. Temperature, humidity and latitude analysis to predict potential spread and seasonality for COVID-19. http://dx.doi.org/10.2139/ssrn.3550308.

[12] Notari. 2020. Temperature dependence of COVID-19 transmission. https://doi.org/10.1101/2020.03.26.20044529.

reporting, as with all of the studies, makes this analysis limited.[13] This study concludes that changes in weather alone will not necessarily lead to declines in cases without extensive public health interventions.

Some limited data support a potential waning of cases in warmer and more humid seasons, yet none are without major limitations. Given that countries currently in "summer" climates, such as Australia and Iran, are experiencing rapid virus spread, a decrease in cases with increases in humidity and temperature elsewhere should not be assumed. Given the lack of immunity to SARS-CoV-2 across the world, if there is an effect of temperature and humidity on transmission, it may not be as apparent as with other respiratory viruses for which there is at least some pre-existing partial immunity. It is useful to note that pandemic influenza strains have not exhibited the typical seasonal pattern of endemic/epidemic strains. There have been 10 influenza pandemics in the past 250-plus years—two started in the northern hemisphere winter, three in the spring, two in the summer, and three in the fall. All had a peak second wave approximately 6 months after emergence of the virus in the human population, regardless of when the initial introduction occurred.

Additional studies as the SARS-CoV-2 pandemic unfolds could shed more light on the effects of climate on transmission.

In summary, although experimental studies show a relationship between higher temperatures and humidity levels, and reduced survival of SARS-CoV-2 in the laboratory, there are many other factors besides environmental temperature, humidity, and survival of the virus outside of the host, that influence and determine transmission rates among humans in the "real world."

My colleagues and I hope this input is helpful to you as you continue to guide the nation's response in this ongoing public health crisis.

Respectfully,
David A. Relman, M.D.
Member
Standing Committee on Emerging Infectious Diseases and 21st Century Health Threats

APPENDIX

Authors and Reviewers of This Rapid Expert Consultation

This rapid expert consultation was prepared by staff of the National Academies of Sciences, Engineering, and Medicine, and members of the National Academies' Standing Committee on Emerging Infectious Diseases and 21st Century Health Threats:

---

[13] Luo et al. 2020. The role of absolute humidity on transmission rates of the COVID-19 outbreak. https://doi.org/10.1101/2020.02.12.20022467.

Kristian Andersen, The Scripps Research Institute; David Relman, Stanford University; and David Walt, Brigham and Women's Hospital and Harvard Medical School.

Harvey Fineberg, chair of the Standing Committee, approved this document. The following individuals served as reviewers: Jim Chappell, Vanderbilt University Medical Center; Mark Denison, Vanderbilt University Medical Center; Michael Diamond, Washington University; Matthew Frieman, University of Maryland School of Medicine; Linsey Marr, Virginia Tech; Michael Osterholm, University of Minnesota; and Stanley Perlman, University of Iowa. Ellen Wright Clayton, Vanderbilt University Medical Center, and Susan Curry, University of Iowa, served as arbiters of this review on behalf of the National Academies' Report Review Committee and their Health and Medicine Division.

Rapid Expert Consultation on SARS-CoV-2 Laboratory Testing for the COVID-19 Pandemic (April 8, 2020)

April 8, 2020

Kelvin Droegemeier, Ph.D.
Office of Science and Technology Policy
Executive Office of the President
Eisenhower Executive Office Building
1650 Pennsylvania Avenue, NW
Washington, DC 20504

Dear Dr. Droegemeier:

Attached please find a rapid expert consultation on the uses, interpretation, and future directions of laboratory tests that was prepared by David Relman, David Walt, and Kristian Andersen, members of the National Academies of Sciences, Engineering, and Medicine's Standing Committee on Emerging Infectious Diseases and 21st Century Health Threats. Details on the authors and reviewers of this rapid expert consultation can be found in the Appendix.

The aim of this rapid expert consultation is to provide scientifically grounded principles that are relevant to decision making about the interpretation of laboratory tests.

This rapid expert consultation covers the current, pertinent studies and points the way to specific research needs in the days and months ahead. We hope this document proves useful to you and your colleagues.

Respectfully,
Harvey V. Fineberg, M.D., Ph.D.
Chair
Standing Committee on Emerging Infectious Diseases and 21st Century Health Threats

This rapid expert consultation responds to your request for information on the interpretation of laboratory tests, future developments, and research needs.

Laboratory confirmation with reliable, standardized testing is the gold standard for determining disease rates. However, especially early after recognition of a new infectious disease, tests with high sensitivity[1] and specificity[2] may not be available that can accurately and consistently separate individuals with the infection from individuals without the infection. It is important to note that clinical judgment, which usually takes into account the probability of infection based on exposure risk and a review of clinical signs and symptoms, is crucial in understanding an infectious disease such as COVID-19 and who may have it.

There are two general types of infectious disease tests—those that detect the disease agent directly (e.g., PCR tests for viral RNA) and those that detect a host response to the disease agent (e.g., serology tests that detect specific antibodies). An increasing number of purveyors now offer COVID-19 tests of each type.

DETECTION OF VIRAL RNA

Most COVID-19 tests in current use detect the disease agent directly and measure viral RNA. Viral RNA indicates current infection and suggests infectivity and transmission risk for others; however, the presence of viral RNA in an individual, especially late in infection, may represent viral remnants rather than intact virus particles capable of transmission. Additional studies on the temporal dynamics of viral RNA in infected persons, across body sites and fluids, and correlations of these measurements with risk of transmission to other individuals, are sorely needed—as is a much greater capacity to perform these tests nationwide.

Current clinical tests for SARS-CoV-2 rely on the detection of viral RNA, using reverse-transcriptase polymerase chain reaction (RT-PCR) or loop-mediated isothermal amplification (LAMP) in nasopharyngeal (NP), oropharyngeal (OP), sputum, or saliva samples. RT-PCR tests have been widely used for the diagnosis of COVID-19. A retrospective study suggested that these tests may be less sensitive in identifying the early phases of disease than computed tomography (CT) scans of the chest, and other clinical and laboratory findings.[3] One study of 51 patients with COVID-19, diagnosed on the basis of a positive RT-PCR at any time during the course of their illness, found that only 35 of the 51 had a positive RT-PCR at the time of clinical presentation, while 50 of the 51 had abnormal CT findings at the time of presentation.[4] Neither this nor other studies we have found pinpoint the reasons for false negative results on initial PCR tests, but the reasons may include stage of illness, lower amounts of virus in certain anatomic sites and in certain patients, and suboptimal sample collection methods.

---

[1] Sensitivity: The probability of a positive test result in a patient who has the disease. An error in sensitivity produces a false negative result.

[2] Specificity: The probability of a negative test result in a patient who does not have the disease. An error in specificity produces a false positive result.

[3] Xu et al. 2020. Analysis and prediction of false negative results for SARS-CoV-2 detection with pharyngeal swab specimen in COVID-19 patients: A retrospective study. https://doi.org/10.1101/2020.03.26.20043042.

[4] Fang et al. 2020. Sensitivity of chest CT for COVID-19: Comparison to RT-PCR. *Radiology*. https://doi.org/10.1148/radiol.2020200432.

LAMP testing methods developed for SARS-CoV in 2004 were found to be more rapid, more simple to perform, and cheaper than conventional methods.[5] LAMP also appears to be sensitive and specific for SARS-CoV-2 when compared to RT-PCR, using spiked non-patient samples.[6] Large cohort studies are now under way to test whether these advantages hold up.

Rapid tests that detect viral RNA include Cepheid's SARS-CoV-2 cartridge[7] for use on its rapid PCR Xpert platform with a 45-minute turn-around, and Abbott's ID NOW COVID-19 isothermal amplification test[8] for use on its ID NOW platform with results in less than 15 minutes. Both of these tests are helpful toward building local capacity, but at the time of this rapid expert consultation (April 8), neither had achieved levels of production that come close to meeting national needs. Their use will be limited to sites that have invested in those instrument platforms; in addition, the robustness of their supply chains has not been adequately confirmed. Rapid tests like these will be most valuable in assessing patients for whom emergency procedures such as surgery, if undertaken without a test result, might pose a high risk of disease transmission.

Although not yet in the clinical workplace, a CRISPR-Cas12 or -Cas13 based diagnostic test for SARS-CoV-2 might offer advantages over current technologies. CRISPR-Cas12 and -Cas13 provide for high sensitivity (can detect as few as 10 gene copies), specificity, portability, easy read-out (e.g., colorimetric with paper strips), speed (~45 minutes), and low cost (few dollars per sample).[9,10,11]

A recent report indicates that viral RNA can be detected by RT-PCR directly in NP swab samples without the need for an RNA extraction step, presumably due to the high burden of infection at this body site and the shedding of viral RNA from dead and lysed host cells.[12] In this report, there was only a 20-fold decrease in sensitivity of viral detection; other reports suggest ~100-fold loss in sensitivity. This is an important finding in the event that current shortages of RNA extraction kits continue or worsen.

One approach for increasing the scale of PCR testing relies on pooling samples for initial screening, with follow-up testing of subsets of the original pool if the initial screen produces a positive result.[13] While early tests of this approach are promising and this

---

[5] Thai et al. 2004. Development and evaluation of a novel loop-mediated isothermal amplification method for rapid detection of severe acute respiratory syndrome coronavirus. *Journal of Clinical Microbioliogy* 42(5):1956-1961.

[6] Lamb et al. 2020. Rapid detection of novel coronavirus (COVID-19) by reverse transcription-loop-mediated isothermal amplification. https://doi.org/10.1101/2020.02.19.20025155.

[7] Cepheid. 2020. Xpert Xpress SARS-CoV-2 has received FDA Emergency Use Authorization. https://www.cepheid.com/coronavirus (accessed April 2, 2020).

[8] Abbott. 2020. Detect COVID-19 in as little as 5 minutes. https://www.abbott.com/corpnewsroom/product-and-innovation/detect-covid-19-in-as-little-as-5-minutes.html (accessed April 2, 2020).

[9] Kellner et al. 2019. SHERLOCK: Nucleic acid detection with CRISPR nucleases. *Nature Protocols* 14:2986-3012.

[10] Lucia et al. 2020. An ultrasensitive, rapid, and portable coronavirus SARS-CoV-2 sequence detection method based on CRISPR-Cas12. https://doi.org/10.1101/2020.02.29.971127.

[11] Metsky et al. 2020. CRISPR-based surveillance for COVID-19 using genomically-comprehensive machine learning design. https://doi.org/10.1101/2020.02.26.967026.

[12] Bruce et al. 2020. RT-qPCR detection of SARS-CoV-2 RNA from patient nasopharyngeal swab using Qiagen RNeasy kits or directly via omission of an RNA extraction step. https://biorxiv.org/content/10.1101/2020.03.20.001008v1 (accessed April 2, 2020).

[13] Yelin et al. 2020. Evaluation of COVID-19 RT-zPCR test in multi-sample pools. https://doi.org/10.1101/2020.03.26.20039438.

type of multiplexing strategy has worked in other disease screening scenarios, it will require further validation. If pooled samples prove feasible, pooling could multiply the throughput of test facilities by 5- or 10-fold, depending on the prevalence of positive results in the sampled population.

DETECTION OF HOST IMMUNE RESPONSE

Tests of the second type (i.e., those that detect a host response to the disease agent) typically measure specific antibodies to the agent, and a number of these so-called serological tests for SARS-CoV-2 are coming online as well. These tests also offer useful information, but the utility and meaning of serological information are quite distinct from the utility and meaning of viral RNA diagnostic test results. Serological tests measure whether an individual has been previously exposed to the agent; however, they have also been used to complement RT-PCR results in establishing a diagnosis later in the course of illness (see also *Rapid Expert Consultation on Viral Shedding and Antibody Response (April 8, 2020)*). IgM antibodies typically appear within days to about a week after the onset of symptoms, and persist for weeks to a month or two. They appear earlier than IgG antibodies but are less specific. IgG antibodies typically first appear in the bloodstream 2 weeks after infection and last for months and in some cases, years. Anti-SARS-CoV-2 antibodies of various types have been detected in COVID-19 patients a median of 5 to 14 days following symptom onset (see also *Rapid Expert Consultation on Viral Shedding and Antibody Response (April 8, 2020)*). Within a few weeks of infection, SARS-CoV-2 antibodies and viral RNA can both be present in the same individual. In general, serological results, especially IgM measurement, may be less specific than molecular tests. All SARS-CoV-2 serological study results should be viewed as suspect until rigorous controls are performed and performance characteristics described, as antibody detection methods can vary considerably, and most so far have not described well-standardized controls. Samples from patients with seasonal (non-SARS-CoV-2) coronavirus infections are especially important as negative controls (see below).

The presence of antibodies against an infectious agent can be a valuable marker for past infection in population-based epidemiologic studies, and they enable assessments of the efficacy of various public interventions in preventing disease spread. Antibodies can also indicate host immunity against the agent. However, in the case of SARS-CoV-2, it is not known whether the presence of antibodies indicates protection from illness.

A consideration of the human immune response to the four seasonal coronaviruses, and to previous emerging coronaviruses, is important to note here. By adulthood, almost everyone has antibodies against common viruses (hCoV-OC43, hCoV-229E, hCoV-HKU1, and hCoV-NL63); however, people still get infected with these viruses each winter. There are limited data on how this happens, what the antibodies in our blood actually recognize on these viruses, why naturally occurring antibodies do not protect us, how the seasonal coronaviruses mutate each year, and why we see them in the winter but not in the summer.

In analyses of antibody responses in individuals exposed to MERS-CoV, commercial ELISA kits in general exhibited good specificity but poor sensitivity compared to a plaque reduction/neutralization titer assay used in a research laboratory.[14] Establishing standards with high sensitivity and specificity that are accepted and followed by all laboratories will be key to determining true exposure to SARS-CoV-2 and potential immunity and for obtaining validated results. In addition, in the case of MERS, as with SARS-CoV-2 (see above), high levels of antibody and of virus are often found in the same patient.[15] Measurements of T cell responses to SARS-CoV-2 may be useful as a complement to antibody assays, in the same fashion as with MERS-CoV.[16]

DETERMINATION OF INFECTIVITY

Current molecular tests for RNA do not determine whether there is viable virus in the specimen. For example, high levels of viral RNA can be found in stool samples, but infectious virus is typically not isolated from these samples.[17] Some types of viral RNA intermediates may be indicative of active replication in, or proximal to, the specimen. These RNAs are produced during the viral life cycle in a human cell but are not incorporated into the mature virus particle; thus, the presence of these RNAs indicates active replication, rather than previously assembled viable virus. The identification and development of assays for these non-packaged replicative RNA intermediates may have clinical utility in predicting an increased likelihood of the presence of infectious virus. Protein-based tests for virus are more likely to be superior in detecting infectivity than genomic tests as proteins are degraded more rapidly than viral RNA.

RESEARCH NEEDS

There are several important unmet needs, some of which are now the subject of ongoing research.

It would be quite helpful to have a test that identifies infected individuals before they are symptomatic <u>and</u> before they shed the virus and become infectious for others. One promising approach is to identify human genes that are expressed early in infection, perhaps in blood or saliva, with some specificity for the infection of interest. Work on broad classes of viral and bacterial infections suggests that this may be possible,[18,19] and groundwork on SARS-CoV-2 has begun.[20]

---

[14] Alshukairi et al. 2018. High prevalence of MERS-CoV infection in camel workers in Saudi Arabia. *mBio* 9(5):e01985-18. DOI: 10.1128/mBio.01985-18.

[15] Corman et al. 2016. Viral shedding and antibody response in 37 patients with Middle East respiratory syndrome coronavirus infection. *Clinical Infectious Diseases* 62(4):477-483. DOI: 10.1093/cid/civ951.

[16] Zhao et al. 2017. Recovery from the Middle East respiratory syndrome is associated with antibody and T cell responses. *Science Immunology* 2:eaan5393. DOI: 10.1126/sciimmunol.aan5393.

[17] Wölfel et al. 2020. Virological assessment of hospitalized patients with COVID-2019. *Nature*. https://doi.org/10.1038/s41586-020-2196-x.

[18] Mayhew et al. 2020. A generalizable 29-mRNA neural-network classifier for acute bacterial and viral infections. *Nature Communications* 11:1177. https://www.nature.com/articles/s41467-020-14975-w (accessed April 4, 2020).

[19] Warsinske et al. 2019. Host-response-based gene signatures for tuberculosis diagnosis: A systematic comparison of 16 signatures. *PLOS Medicine* 16(4):e1002786. DOI: 10.1371/journal.pmed.1002786.

[20] Blanco-Melo et al. 2020. SARS-CoV-2 launches a unique transcriptional signature from in vitro, ex vivo, and in vivo systems. https://doi.org/10.1101/2020.03.24.004655.

A comprehensive mapping of antibody specificity during the course of SARS-CoV-2 infection (i.e., a survey of antibody reactivity and function) would greatly help in understanding variability in the outcome of infection in different individuals, risk stratification, the relationship of pre-existing antibody profiles with SARS-CoV-2 outcome, and the identification of optimal vaccine antigens. An interesting preprint by Khan et al. describes the creation of a microarray with 67 antigens from all known coronaviruses and other known respiratory viruses that will help elucidate whether baseline anti-coronavirus antibodies might influence the clinical course of COVID-19 and help to describe the evolution of the immune response during the course of SARS-CoV-2 infection.[21] Other, more comprehensive antibody profiling technology already exists, and awaits application to COVID-19 patient serum samples.[22]

Well-controlled longitudinal studies are critically needed as they can determine the relationship between different types of SARS-CoV-2-specific antibodies and the likelihood of an individual becoming re-infected. A critical goal is identification of antibodies that neutralize and block SARS-CoV-2 viral infection, as well as the determination of how much neutralizing antibody is needed for protection. As a technical note, proper identification of neutralizing antibodies will require not only pseudotyped virus with the appropriate epitopes, but fresh clinical isolates of SARS-CoV-2 as well.

SUMMARY

The two general classes of diagnostic tests, one to detect viral RNA and the other to detect human antibodies directed against the virus, each provide a distinct set of benefits and weaknesses. Detection of viral RNA generally indicates active, ongoing infection and suggests infectiousness for others, especially early in the course of infection, although the persistence of detectable viral RNA weeks after infection may no longer be synonymous with a virus capable of causing infection. Antibody tests provide evidence of past exposure and possible immunity; however, the relationship between antibody and protection has not been established for this virus. Both types of tests will require proper validation and new longitudinal studies of infected individuals before they can be properly interpreted.

My colleagues and I hope this input is helpful to you as you continue to guide the nation's response in this ongoing public health crisis.

Respectfully,
David A. Relman, M.D.
Member
Standing Committee on Emerging Infectious Diseases and 21st Century Health Threats

---

[21] Khan et al. 2020. Analysis of serological cross-reactivity between common human coronaviruses and SARS-CoV-2 using coronavirus antigen microarray. https://doi.org/10.1101/2020.03.24.006544.

[22] Xu et al. 2015. Comprehensive serological profiling of human populations using a synthetic human virome. *Science* 348(6239):aaa0698. DOI: 10.1126/science.aaa0698.

APPENDIX

Authors and Reviewers of This Rapid Expert Consultation

This rapid expert consultation was prepared by staff of the National Academies of Sciences, Engineering, and Medicine, and members of the National Academies' Standing Committee on Emerging Infectious Diseases and 21st Century Health Threats: Kristian Andersen, The Scripps Research Institute; David Relman, Stanford University; and David Walt, Brigham and Women's Hospital and Harvard Medical School.

Harvey Fineberg, chair of the Standing Committee, approved this document. The following individuals served as reviewers: Jim Chappell, Vanderbilt University Medical Center; Mark Denison, Vanderbilt University Medical Center; Michael Diamond, Washington University; Matthew Frieman, University of Maryland School of Medicine; Linsey Marr, Virginia Tech; Michael Osterholm, University of Minnesota; and Stanley Perlman, University of Iowa. Ellen Wright Clayton, Vanderbilt University Medical Center, and Susan Curry, University of Iowa, served as arbiters of this review on behalf of the National Academies' Report Review Committee and their Health and Medicine Division.

Rapid Expert Consultation on the Effectiveness of Fabric Masks for the COVID-19 Pandemic (April 8, 2020)

April 8, 2020

Kelvin Droegemeier, Ph.D.
Office of Science and Technology Policy
Executive Office of the President
Eisenhower Executive Office Building
1650 Pennsylvania Avenue, NW
Washington, DC 20504

Dear Dr. Droegemeier:

Attached please find a rapid expert consultation that was prepared by Rich Besser and Baruch Fischhoff, members of the National Academies of Sciences, Engineering, and Medicine's Standing Committee on Emerging Infectious Diseases and 21st Century Health Threats, with input from Sundaresan Jayaraman and Michael Osterholm. Details on the authors and reviewers of this rapid expert consultation can be found in the Appendix.

The aim of this rapid expert consultation is to respond to your request concerning the effectiveness of homemade fabric masks worn by the general public to protect others, as distinct from protecting the wearer. The request stems from an interest in reducing transmission within the community by individuals who are infected, potentially contagious, but asymptomatic.

Overall, the available evidence is inconclusive about the degree to which homemade fabric masks may suppress the spread of infection from the wearer to others. For as long as homemade fabric masks are in use by the public, the investigations outlined at the end of the rapid expert consultation could reduce uncertainty about the effectiveness of these masks.

My colleagues and I hope this input is helpful to you as you continue to guide the nation's response in this ongoing public health crisis.

Respectfully,
Harvey V. Fineberg, M.D., Ph.D.
Chair
Standing Committee on Emerging Infectious Diseases and 21st Century Health Threats

This rapid expert consultation responds to your request concerning the effectiveness of homemade fabric masks worn by the general public to protect others, as distinct from protecting the wearer. The request stems from an interest in reducing transmission within the community by individuals who are infected, potentially contagious, but asymptomatic or presymptomatic. As discussed below, the answer depends on both the masks themselves and how infected individuals use them.

The following analysis is restricted to the effectiveness of homemade fabric masks, of the sort illustrated in recommendations[1] directed at the general public, in terms of their ability to reduce viral spread during the asymptomatic or presymptomatic period. It does not apply to either N95 respirators or medical masks.

In considering the evidence about the potential effectiveness of homemade fabric masks, it is important to bear in mind how a respiratory virus such as SARS-CoV-2 spreads from person to person. Current research supports the possibility that, in addition to being spread by respiratory droplets that one can see and feel, SARS-CoV-2 can also be spread by invisible droplets, as small as 5 microns (or micrometers), and by even smaller bioaerosol particles.[2] Such tiny bioaerosol particles may be found in an infected person's normal exhalation.[3] The relative contribution of each particle size in disease transmission is unknown.

There is limited research on the efficacy of fabric masks for influenza and specifically for SARS-CoV-2. As we describe below, the few available experimental studies

---

[1] Centers for Disease Control and Prevention (CDC) Recommendation Regarding the Use of Cloth Face Coverings, Especially in Areas of Significant Community-Based Transmission in response to COVID-19. https://www.cdc.gov/coronavirus/2019-ncov/prevent-getting-sick/cloth-face-cover.html.

[2] Gralton et al. (2011) noted the following in regard to particulate size and the importance of airborne precautions whenever there is a risk of both droplet and aerosol transmission: "Regardless of the complexities and limitations of sizing particles and the contention of size cut-offs, it remains that particles have been observed to occupy a size range between 0.05 and 500 microns. Even using the conservative cut-off of 10 microns, rather than the 5 micron to define between airborne and droplet transmission, this size range indicates that particles do not exclusively disperse by airborne transmission or via droplet transmission but rather avail of both methods simultaneously. This suggestion is further supported by the simultaneous detection of both large and small particles. In line with these observations and logic, current dichotomous infection control precautions should be updated to include measures to contain both modes of aerosolised transmission. This may require airborne precautions to be used when at risk of any aerosolized infection, as airborne precautions are considered as a step-up from droplet precautions." Gralton et al. 2011. The role of particle size in aerosolised pathogen transmission: A review. *Journal of Infection* 62(1):1-13. DOI: 10.1016/j.jinf.2010.11.010.

[3] National Academies of Sciences, Engineering, and Medicine. 2020. *Rapid Expert Consultation on the Possibility of Bioaerosol Spread of SARS-CoV-2 for the COVID-19 Pandemic (April 1, 2020)*. Washington, DC: The National Academies Press. https://doi.org/10.17226/25769.

have important limitations in their relevance and methods. Any type of mask will have its own capacity to arrest particles of different sizes. Even if the filtering capacity of a mask were well understood, however, the degree to which it could in practice reduce disease spread depends on the unknown role of each particle size in transmission.

Asymptomatic but infected individuals are of special concern, and the particles they would emit from breathing are predominantly bioaerosols. To complicate matters further, different individuals vary in the extent to which they emit bioaerosols while breathing. Because of the concern with spread from asymptomatic individuals, who, unlike symptomatic persons, may be out and about, this rapid expert consultation includes the effects of fabric masks on bioaerosol transmission.

IMPACT OF MASK DESIGN AND FABRICATION ON PERFORMANCE

Any effects of fabric masks will depend on how and how well they are made. In an unpublished study whose raw data are not currently available, Jayaraman et al.[4] examined a range of fabric-based filtration systems, in terms of how well they stopped particles (filtration efficiency) and how much they impeded breathing (differential pressure, Delta-P, the measured pressure drop across the material, which determines the resistance of the material to air flow).[5] The study varied fabric type (woven, woven brushed, knitted, knitted brushed, knitted pile), material type (cotton, polyester, polypropylene, silk), fabric parameters (fabric areal density, yarn linear density, fabric weight), and construction type (number of layers, orientation of the layers). The study found wide variation in filtration efficiency. A mask made from a four-layer woven handkerchief fabric, of a sort that might be found in many homes, had 0.7% filtration efficiency for 0.3 micron size particles and a Delta-P of 0.1". Much higher filtration efficiency was observed with filters created specifically for the research from a five-layer woven brushed fabric (35.3% of the particles were trapped) and from four layers of polyester knitted cut-pile fabric (50% of the particles were trapped with a Delta-P of 0.2").

The greater a mask's breathing resistance, which is reflected in a higher Delta-P, the more difficult it is for users to wear it consistently, and the more likely they are to experience breathing difficulties when they do.[6] Although Jayaraman et al. did not measure breathing resistance directly, almost all of the masks they tested would be expected to have breathing resistance within the range of commercial N95 respirators. One mask that used 16 layers of the handkerchief fabric, in order to increase filtration efficiency (63% efficiency with a Delta-P of 0.425"), had breathing resistance greater

---

[4] Jayaraman et al. *Pandemic Flu—Textile Solutions Pilot: Design and Development of Innovative Medical Masks*, Final Technical Report, Georgia Institute of Technology, Atlanta, Georgia, submitted to CDC, February 14, 2012.

[5] The tests were conducted according to ASTM F2299-3 test method using poly-dispersed sodium chloride aerosol particles with an airflow rate of 30L/min and airflow velocity of 11 cm/s. Aerosol sizes measured: 0.1, 0.2, 0.3, 0.4, 0.5, 0.7, 1, and 2 microns.

[6] 3M™ Health Care Particulate Respirator and Surgical Masks, Healthcare Respirator Brochure, 3M Company, Minnesota.

than that of commercial N95 respirators, which would cause great discomfort to many wearers and cause some to pass out.

An additional consideration in the effectiveness of any mask is how well it fits the user.[7] Even with the best material, if a mask does not fit, virus-containing particles can escape through creases and gaps between the mask and face. Leakage can also occur if the holding mechanism (e.g., straps, Velcro®) is weak. We found no studies of non-expert individuals' ability to produce properly fitting masks. Nor did we find any studies of the effectiveness of masks produced by professionals, when following instructions available to the general public (e.g., online). Given the current Centers for Disease Control and Prevention (CDC) recommendation to wear cloth face coverings in public settings in areas of significant community-based transmission, additional research should examine the ability of the general public to produce properly fitted fabric masks when following communications and instructions.

ROLE OF THE WEARER

The effectiveness of homemade fabric masks will also depend on the wearer's behavior. Even if a mask could fit well, its effectiveness still depends on how well the wearer puts it on and keeps it in place. As mentioned, breathing difficulty can impede effective use (e.g., pulling a mask down), as can moisture from the wearer's breath. Moisture saturation is inevitable with fabrics available in most homes. Moreover, moisture can trap the virus and become a potential contamination source for others after a mask is removed.

EFFECTIVENESS OF HOMEMADE FABRIC MASKS IN PROTECTING OTHERS

Several experimental studies have examined the effects of fabric masks on the transmission of droplets of various sizes.

Anfinrud et al.[8] shared via email that they used sensitive laser light-scattering procedures to detect droplet emission while people were speaking. The authors found that "a damp homemade cloth facemask" reduced droplet emission to background levels (when users said "Stay Healthy" three times). However, when a fabric is dampened, the yarns can swell over time, potentially altering its filtering performance. That swelling will depend on the fabric: cotton swells readily, synthetics less so. In an unpublished follow-up experiment, Anfinrud et al. repeated their study with a variety of dry (not moistened) cloths, including a standard workers dust mask (not certified N95) and a

---

[7] Davies et al. (2013) noted that, "Although any material may provide a physical barrier to an infection, if as a mask it does not fit well around the nose and mouth, or the material freely allows infectious aerosols to pass through it, then it will be of no benefit." Davies et al. 2013. Testing the efficacy of homemade masks: Would they protect in an influenza pandemic? *Disaster Medicine and Public Health Preparedness* 7(4):413-418. DOI: 10.1017/dmp.2013.43.

[8] Anfinrud et al. In Press. Could SARS-CoV-2 be transmitted via speech droplets? *New England Journal of Medicine*. https://doi.org/10.1101/2020.04.02.20051177.

mask rigged from an airline eye covering. They found that all of these masks reduced droplet emission generated by speech to background level.[9]

Bae et al. (2020) evaluated the effectiveness of surgical and cotton masks in filtering SARS-CoV-2.[10] They found that neither kind of mask reduced the dissemination of SARS-CoV-2 from the coughs of four symptomatic patients with COVID-19 to the environment and external mask surface. The study used disposable surgical masks (180 mm × 90 mm, 3 layers [inner surface mixed with polypropylene and polyethylene, polypropylene filter, and polypropylene outer surface], pleated, bulk packaged in cardboard; KM Dental Mask, KM Healthcare Corp) and reusable 100% cotton masks (160 mm × 135 mm, 2 layers, individually packaged in plastic; Seoulsa). The median viral loads of nasopharyngeal and saliva samples from the four participants were 5.66 log copies/mL and 4.00 log copies/mL, respectively. The median viral loads after coughs without a mask, with a surgical mask, and with a cotton mask were similar: 2.56 log copies/mL, 2.42 log copies/mL, and 1.85 log copies/mL, respectively. All swabs from the outer mask surfaces of the masks were positive for SARS-CoV-2, whereas swabs from three out of the four symptomatic patients from the inner mask surfaces were negative. Note that this study focused on symptomatic patients who coughed.

Rengasamy et al. (2010)[11] tested the filtration performance of five common household fabric materials: sweatshirts, T-shirts, towels, scarves, and cloth masks (of unknown material) in a laboratory setting. These fabric materials were tested for sprays having both similar and diverse particle sizes (monodisperse and polydisperse). The range of sizes used in the study (0.02-1 micron) includes that of potential virus-containing droplets.[12] The study projected the particles at face velocities, typical of breathing at rest and during exertion (5.5 and 16.5 cm/s). The test also examined N95 respirator filter media. At the lower velocity, 0.12% of particles penetrated the N95 respirator material; at the higher velocity, penetration was less than 5%. For the five common household fabric materials, across the tests, penetration ranged from about 40-90%, indicating a 10-60% reduction. The authors concluded that common fabric materials may provide a low level of protection against nanoparticles, including those in the size ranges of virus-containing particles in exhaled breath (0.02-1 micron). However, Gralton et al. (2011) found particles generated from respiratory activities range from 0.01 up to 500 microns, with a particle size range of 0.05 to 500 microns associated with infection. They stress the need for airborne precautions to be used when at risk of any aerosolized infection, as airborne precautions are considered as a step-up from droplet precautions.

---

[9] Personal communication, Adriaan Bax, National Institutes of Health, April 4, 2020.

[10] Bae et al. 2020. Effectiveness of surgical and cotton masks in blocking SARS-CoV-2: A controlled comparison in 4 patients. *Annals of Internal Medicine*. DOI: 10.7326/M20-1342.

[11] Rengasamy et al. 2010. Simple respiratory protection—evaluation of the filtration performance of cloth masks and common fabric materials against 20-1000 nm size particles. *Annals of Occupational Hygiene* 54(7):789-798. https://doi.org/10.1093/annhyg/meq044.

[12] According to Gralton et al. (2011), particles generated from respiratory activities range from 0.01 up to 500 microns, with a particle size range of 0.05 to 500 microns associated with infection. Gralton et al. 2011. The role of particle size in aerosolised pathogen transmission: A review. *Journal of Infection* 62:1-13. DOI: 10.1016/j.jinf.2010.11.010.

Davies et al. (2013)[13] had 21 healthy volunteers make their own face masks from fresh, unworn cotton t-shirts. This is the only study we found with user-made masks. Participants then coughed into a box, when wearing their own mask, a surgical mask, or no mask. They received no help or guidance from the researcher in making or fitting their masks. The researchers took samples of particles settling onto agar plates and a Casella slit sampler in the box. Under the baseline conditions of no mask, only a small number of colony-forming units (indicative of bacteria) were detected, limiting the opportunity to demonstrate reductions. Still, the investigators reported that both homemade and surgical masks reduced the number of large-sized microorganisms expelled by volunteers, with the surgical mask being more effective.

van der Sande et al. (2008)[14] examined the extent to which respirator masks, surgical masks, and tea-cloth masks made by the researchers would reduce tiny (0.02-1 micron) particle counts on one side of the mask compared to the other. They used burning candles in a test room to generate particles. Two of the study's three experiments examined the protection afforded the wearer (reduced particle counts inside the masks compared to outside). Although not directly germane to the question of protecting others, the study found a modest degree of protection for the wearer from cloth masks, an intermediate degree from surgical masks, and a marked degree with the equivalent of N95 masks. For example, among adults, N95 masks provided 25 times the protection of surgical masks and 50 times the protection of cloth masks. The study's third experiment tested the effectiveness of the three masks at reducing emissions from a simulation dummy head that produced uniform "exhalations." It found that cloth masks reduced emitted particles (leakage) by one-fifth, surgical masks reduced it by one-half, and N95-equivalent masks reduced it by two-thirds.

MacIntyre et al. (2015)[15] conducted a randomized controlled trial comparing infection rates of 1,607 hospital health care workers wearing cloth (two layers, made of cotton) or medical masks (three layers, made of non-woven material) while performing their normal tasks. Workers who used cloth masks experienced much higher rates of influenza-like illness (relative risk = 13.00, 95% confidence interval 1.59 to 100.07). This study measured the protective effect for the wearer, rather than the protection of others from the wearer, and did not include a condition with individuals wearing no masks.

EFFECT ON USERS' RISK BEHAVIOR

In our rapid review, we found no studies of the effects of wearing masks on users' behavior. Speculatively, for some users, masks could provide a constant reminder of the importance of social distancing, as well as signal its importance to others, strengthening the social norm of social distancing. Conversely, for some users, masks might "crowd out" other precautionary behaviors, giving them a feeling that they have done enough to protect themselves and others. Prior research, conducted in less intense settings,

---

[13] Davies et al. 2013. Testing the efficacy of homemade masks: Would they protect in an influenza pandemic? *Disaster Medicine and Public Health Preparedness* 7(4):413-418. DOI: 10.1017/dmp.2013.43.

[14] van der Sande et al. 2008. Professional and home-made face masks reduce exposure to respiratory infections among the general population. *PLOS ONE* 3(7):e2618. DOI: 10.1371/journal.pone.0002618.

[15] MacIntyre et al. 2015. A cluster randomised trial of cloth masks compared with medical masks in healthcare workers. *BMJ Open* 5(4):e006577. DOI: 10.1136/bmjopen-2014-006577.

could support either speculation. Focused research could help determine when precautionary behaviors reinforce or displace one another.

It is critically important that any discussion of homemade fabric masks reinforce the central importance of physical distancing and personal hygiene (frequent handwashing) in reducing spread of infection.

CONCLUSIONS

There are no studies of individuals wearing homemade fabric masks in the course of their typical activities. Therefore, we have only limited, indirect evidence regarding the effectiveness of such masks for protecting others, when made and worn by the general public on a regular basis. That evidence comes primarily from laboratory studies testing the effectiveness of different materials at capturing particles of different sizes.

The evidence from these laboratory filtration studies suggests that such fabric masks may reduce the transmission of larger respiratory droplets. There is little evidence regarding the transmission of small aerosolized particulates of the size potentially exhaled by asymptomatic or presymptomatic individuals with COVID-19. The extent of any protection will depend on how the masks are made and used. It will also depend on how mask use affects users' other precautionary behaviors, including their use of better masks, when those become widely available. Those behavioral effects may undermine or enhance homemade fabric masks' overall effect on public health. The current level of benefit, if any, is not possible to assess.

Research could provide firmer answers by assessing the effectiveness of such fabric masks, as made and used by the general public. That research would have the goals of providing the public with (1) usable instructions on how to make, fit, use, and clean homemade fabric masks; (2) estimates of the protection that such masks afford users and others in different environments (e.g., where the likelihood of contact is higher, like grocery stores, compared to wearing masks all of the time); and (3) effective reinforcement of other precautionary behaviors. That research could provide policy makers with estimates of the net effect of encouraging the use of homemade fabric masks on public health, with realistic estimates of how such masks will be made and used, as well as how they will affect other precautionary behaviors of users and others who observe and interact with them.

My colleagues and I hope this input is helpful to you as you continue to guide the nation's response in this ongoing public health crisis.

Respectfully,
Richard Besser, M.D.
Member
Standing Committee on Emerging Infectious Diseases and 21st Century Health Threats

Baruch Fischhoff, Ph.D.
Member
Standing Committee on Emerging Infectious Diseases and 21st Century Health Threats

APPENDIX

Authors and Reviewers of This Rapid Expert Consultation

This rapid expert consultation was prepared by staff of the National Academies of Sciences, Engineering, and Medicine, and members of the National Academies' Standing Committee on Emerging Infectious Diseases and 21st Century Health Threats: Richard Besser, Robert Wood Johnson Foundation, and Baruch Fischhoff, Carnegie Mellon University. The following subject-matter experts also provided input: Sundaresan Jayaraman, Georgia Tech, and Michael Osterholm, University of Minnesota.

Harvey Fineberg, chair of the Standing Committee, approved this document. The following individuals served as reviewers: Ned Calonge, The Colorado Trust; Robert Hornik, University of Pennsylvania; Thomas Inglesby, Johns Hopkins Bloomberg School of Public Health Center for Health Security; and Grace Lee, Stanford University. Bobbie A. Berkowitz, Columbia University School of Nursing; Ellen Wright Clayton, Vanderbilt University Medical Center; and Susan Curry, University of Iowa, served as arbiters of this review on behalf of the National Academies' Report Review Committee and their Health and Medicine Division.

Rapid Expert Consultation on SARS-CoV-2 Viral Shedding and Antibody Response for the COVID-19 Pandemic (April 8, 2020)

April 8, 2020

Kelvin Droegemeier, Ph.D.
Office of Science and Technology Policy
Executive Office of the President
Eisenhower Executive Office Building
1650 Pennsylvania Avenue, NW
Washington, DC 20504

Dear Dr. Droegemeier:

Attached please find a rapid expert consultation in response to your request concerning (1) the duration of viral shedding by stage of infection, clinical signs and symptoms, and patient attributes; (2) the levels and duration of antibody response and related resistance to illness; and (3) the optimal duration of isolation of cases.

Members of the National Academies of Sciences, Engineering, and Medicine's Standing Committee on Emerging Infectious Diseases and 21st Century Health Threats who were instrumental in preparing this response include Peter Daszak, EcoHealth Alliance; Diane E. Griffin, Johns Hopkins Bloomberg School of Public Health; Kent E. Kester, Sanofi Pasteur; and Mark S. Smolinski, Ending Pandemics.

This document stresses what is known and what are the most salient questions yet to be answered to guide critical decisions related to the duration of isolation of infected patients, the potential effectiveness of a vaccine, and when we can be confident that previously infected patients are resistant to re-infection.

My colleagues and I hope this input is helpful to you as you continue to guide the nation's response in this ongoing public health crisis.

Respectfully,
Harvey V. Fineberg, M.D., Ph.D.
Chair
Standing Committee on Emerging Infectious Diseases and 21st Century Health Threats

This rapid expert consultation responds to your request concerning (1) the duration of viral shedding by stage of infection, clinical signs and symptoms, and patient attributes; (2) the levels and duration of antibody response and related resistance to illness; and (3) the optimal duration of isolation of cases.

Our intent is to answer three questions in response to each issue:

- What is the relevant scientific evidence and state of current scientific knowledge?
- Who is doing the best work in the area and what new results can we anticipate?
- Gaps in knowledge: What investigations should be initiated or extended to provide a more complete answer?

Shedding of infectious virus from the respiratory tract tends to be highest early in disease. This is followed by a prolonged period of viral RNA shedding, but the extent to which this represents infectious virus is uncertain.[1] In addition, the role of shedding from the gastrointestinal tract in transmission is unclear. Antibody responses begin to appear over a period of days to weeks after infection. Studies of SARS and MERS survivors suggest that antibody responses for SARS-CoV-1 and MERS-CoV are not durable.[2,3,4] Further investigation is needed to understand the duration of protective immunity for SARS-CoV-2. The groups referenced in this rapid expert consultation are continuing to produce work in these areas. We anticipate that additional studies based on cases coming out of the United States and Europe will provide further information on these critical topics.

(1) The duration of viral shedding by stage of infection, clinical signs and symptoms, and patient attributes.

Viral shedding has been assessed and detected by culture, but most often by reverse-transcriptase polymerase chain reaction (RT-PCR) for viral RNA.[5] RNA can be detected from infectious virus or from remnants of virus that are no longer infectious. In a patient recovering from an illness who was previously PCR positive, at least two sequential

---

[1] Joynt and Wu. 2020. Understanding COVID-19: What does viral RNA load really mean? *The Lancet Infectious Diseases*. https://doi.org/10.1016/S1473-3099(20)30237-1.

[2] Alshukairi et al. 2016. Antibody response and disease severity in healthcare worker MERS survivors. *Emerging Infectious Diseases* 22(6):1113-1115. https://dx.doi.org/10.3201/eid2206.160010.

[3] Liu et al. 2006. Two-year prospective study of the humoral immune response of patients with severe acute respiratory syndrome. *The Journal of Infectious Diseases* 193(6):792-795.

[4] Wu et al. 2007. Duration of antibody responses after severe acute respiratory syndrome. *Emerging Infectious Diseases* 13(10):1562-1564. DOI: 10.3201/eid1310.070576.

[5] Wölfel et al. 2020. Virological assessment of hospitalized patients with COVID-2019. *Nature*. https://doi.org/10.1038/s41586-020-2196-x.

negative tests for viral RNA is a reasonable indicator of when infectious virus is no longer being shed. Most studies have analyzed respiratory secretions (throat and/or nasopharyngeal samples), but stool samples are also often positive for RNA later in the course of the infection while other sites (e.g., blood, urine, tears, vaginal secretions) are usually negative. These data are likely to be important for the understanding of routes and periods of transmission.

It is not uncommon for viral shedding in respiratory secretions to occur 2-3 days prior to first symptoms.[6,7,8] Higher amounts of virus and viral RNA are seen early in infection independent of severity of symptoms with sputum and nasopharyngeal samples more likely to be positive than throat swab samples.[9,10,11,12,13] More severe clinical disease is associated with longer persistence of viral RNA shedding and may represent a significant occupational transmission risk for health care workers.[14,15] Viral RNA shedding for up to a week after the resolution of symptoms is common and in one case has been documented to continue for as long as 49 days although this viral RNA may not represent infectious virus.[16,17,18,19] No differences in these parameters have been detected based on age or sex.

In addition, gastrointestinal symptoms may be common and viral RNA is frequently detected in stool. Viral RNA persists in stool after symptoms have subsided for longer

---

[6] He. 2020. Temporal dynamics in viral shedding and transmissibility of COVID-19. *medRxiv*.

[7] Kimball et al. 2020. Asymptomatic and presymptomatic SARS-CoV-2 infections in residents of a long-term care skilled nursing facility—King County, Washington, March 2020. *Morbidity and Mortality Weekly Report* 69(13):377-381. http://dx.doi.org/10.15585/mmwr.mm6913e1.

[8] Li et al. 2020. Asymptomatic and human-to-human transmission of SARS-CoV-2 in a 2-family cluster, Xuzhou, China. *Emerging Infectious Diseases* 26(7). https://doi.org/10.3201/eid2607.200718.

[9] Wölfel et al. 2020. Virological assessment of hospitalized patients with COVID-2019. *Nature*. https://doi.org/10.1038/s41586-020-2196-x.

[10] He. 2020. Temporal dynamics in viral shedding and transmissibility of COVID-19. *medRxiv*.

[11] Yu et al. 2020. Quantitative detection and viral load analysis of SARS-CoV-2 in infected patients. *Clinical Infectious Diseases*. https://doi.org/10.1093/cid/ciaa345.

[12] Zou et al. 2020. SARS-CoV-2 viral load in upper respiratory specimens of infected patients. *New England Journal of Medicine* 382(12):1177-1179. DOI: 10.1056/NEJMc2001737.

[13] Cereda et al. 2020. The early phase of the COVID-19 outbreak in Lombardy, Italy. *medRxiv*.

[14] Liu et al. 2020. Viral dynamics in mild and severe cases of COVID-19. *The Lancet Infectious Diseases*. https://doi.org/10.1016/S1473-3099(20)30232-2.

[15] Lescure et al. 2020. Clinical and virological data of the first cases of COVID-19 in Europe: A case series. *The Lancet Infectious Diseases*. https://doi.org/10.1016/S1473-3099(20)30200-0.

[16] Wölfel et al. 2020. Virological assessment of hospitalized patients with COVID-2019. *Nature*. https://doi.org/10.1038/s41586-020-2196-x.

[17] Zhou et al. 2020. Clinical course and risk factors for mortality of adult inpatients with COVID-19 in Wuhan, China: A retrospective cohort study. *The Lancet* 395(10229):1054-1062. https://doi.org/10.1016/S0140-6736(20)30566-3.

[18] Tan. 2020. Viral kinetics and antibody responses in patients with COVID-19. *medRxiv*.

[19] Young et al. 2020. Epidemiologic features and clinical course of patients infected with SARS-CoV-2 in Singapore. *JAMA* 323(15):1488-1494. DOI: 10.1001/jama.2020.3204.

than in samples from the respiratory tract, but a role in transmission is unclear.[20,21,22,23,24] In a recent report infectious virus was readily isolated from respiratory samples, but not from stool samples.[25]

Gaps in knowledge:

- Effect of various treatments on length of shedding.
- Epidemiologic evidence of transmission while RT-PCR positive after recovery.
- Significance of viral RNA shedding after resolution of symptoms.
- Importance of shedding from non-respiratory sites.
- Innovative assays to determine if the virus is infectious.

(2) Levels and duration of antibody response and related resistance to illness.

The time of antibody detection after infection is dependent on the sensitivity of the assay and the viral protein used as antigen. IgM can be detected by enzyme immunoassay to nucleoprotein 3-6 (median 5) days after onset of symptoms and has been used to complement RT-PCR for diagnosis of COVID-19.[26,27] IgG to the same protein is detected 10-18 (median 14) days after the onset of symptoms.[28] Anti-nucleoprotein antibody did not correlate with virus clearance[29] and a higher antibody titer was independently associated with more severe disease.[30] Antibody to the receptor-binding domain of the

---

[20] Zhang et al. 2020. Molecular and serological investigation of 2019-nCoV infected patients: Implication of multiple shedding routes. *Emerging Microbes & Infections* 9(1):386-389. DOI: 10.1080/22221751.2020.1729071.

[21] Lo et al. 2020. Evaluation of SARS-CoV-2 RNA shedding in clinical specimens and clinical characteristics of 10 patients with COVID-19 in Macau. *International Journal of Biological Sciences* 16(10):1698-1707. DOI: 10.7150/ijbs.45357.

[22] Ling et al. 2020. Persistence and clearance of viral RNA in 2019 novel coronavirus disease rehabilitation patients. *Chinese Medical Journal (English)*. DOI: 10.1097/CM9.0000000000000774.

[23] Xu. 2020. Characteristics of pediatric SARS-CoV-2 infection and potential evidence for persistent fecal viral shedding. *Nature Medicine* 26:502-505. https://doi.org/10.1038/s41591-020-0817-4.

[24] During the SARS epidemic in Hong Kong in 2003, the virus was spread in an apartment complex (Amoy Gardens) due to aerosolized waste flushed from toilets that found its way into the air of other apartments through poorly designed bathroom floor drains.

[25] Wölfel et al. 2020. Virological assessment of hospitalized patients with COVID-2019. *Nature*. https://doi.org/10.1038/s41586-020-2196-x.

[26] Guo et al. 2020. Profiling early humoral response to diagnose novel coronavirus disease (COVID-19). *Clinical Infectious Diseases*. https://doi.org/10.1093/cid/ciaa310.

[27] Zhao et al. 2020. Antibody responses to SARS-CoV-2 in patients of novel coronavirus disease 2019. *Clinical Infectious Diseases*. DOI: 10.1093/cid/ciaa344.

[28] Guo et al. 2020. Profiling early humoral response to diagnose novel coronavirus disease (COVID-19). *Clinical Infectious Diseases*. https://doi.org/10.1093/cid/ciaa310.

[29] Tan. 2020. Viral kinetics and antibody responses in patients with COVID-19. *medRxiv*.

[30] Guo et al. 2020. Profiling early humoral response to diagnose novel coronavirus disease (COVID-19). *Clinical Infectious Diseases*. https://doi.org/10.1093/cid/ciaa310.

spike protein was detected a median of 11 days after the onset of symptoms, but the timing of seroconversion did not correlate with clinical course.[31,32]

The duration of the antibody response and acquired immunity to re-infection will be critical to understanding (1) how effective vaccination is likely to be; (2) how durable immunity is; (3) whether it is possible to achieve herd immunity against COVID-19; and (4) how safe it is for people who are positive in a serology test to return to work. One key uncertainty arises from the fact that we are early in the outbreak and survivors from the first weeks of infection in China are, at most, only 3 months since recovery. Some lessons may be gleaned from evidence about the duration of antibody responses to SARS-CoV and MERS-CoV, which are related viruses. Studies of patients who recovered from the SARS outbreak in 2003 show a steady decrease in amounts of antiviral binding IgG over time with 12% negative at 2 years and 50% at 3 years.[33,34] Similarly, health care workers with mild to moderate MERS-CoV infection had no detectable antiviral binding IgG 18 months after recovery.[35] The response to SARS-CoV-2 is likely to be similar to this closely related virus. Longitudinal data from the large numbers of recovered cases in China from earlier in the outbreak may give us insight into the temporal dynamics of antibody titers to this virus.

Gaps in knowledge:

- Evaluation of whether the presence of antibodies confers protection from illness due to re-infection, and if so, what levels of antibodies are needed.
- A better understanding of the role of specific antibodies will inform possible therapy with immune plasma and the development of monoclonal antibodies for potential treatment, as well as vaccine design.
- Following antibody titers in cohorts of patients with mild, moderate, severe, and critical COVID-19 disease will be revealing. This would best be done in multiple geographies, with diverse age classes, ethnic background, etc.
- Evidence of waning antibody titer can be anticipated after 2 years, but any indication of earlier significant drop in titers per age class or other grouping would be very important to identify because it might affect vaccine efficacy, the ability of these people to be re-infected and the potential for disease attenuation with an anamnestic response.

---

[31] Wölfel et al. 2020. Virological assessment of hospitalized patients with COVID-2019. *Nature*. https://doi.org/10.1038/s41586-020-2196-x.

[32] Zhao et al. 2020. Antibody responses to SARS-CoV-2 in patients of novel coronavirus disease 2019. *Clinical Infectious Diseases*. DOI: 10.1093/cid/ciaa344.

[33] Liu et al. 2006. Two-year prospective study of the humoral immune response of patients with severe acute respiratory syndrome. *The Journal of Infectious Diseases* 193(6):792-795.

[34] Wu et al. 2007. Duration of antibody responses after severe acute respiratory syndrome. *Emerging Infectious Diseases* 13(10):1562-1564. DOI: 10.3201/eid1310.070576.

[35] Alshukairi et al. 2016. Antibody response and disease severity in healthcare worker MERS survivors. *Emerging Infectious Diseases* 22(6):1113-1115. https://dx.doi.org/10.3201/eid2206.160010.

(3) Optimal duration of isolation of cases.

Because many patients continue to be RT-PCR positive for viral RNA in both respiratory secretions and stool, this is a difficult question that will best be informed by observational studies of transmission from discharged patients with known status for viral RNA by RT-PCR. Waiting for all tests to be repeatedly negative is the most conservative approach, but may result in prolonged unnecessary isolation. Assessment of humoral and cellular immune response may also be informative. Current Centers for Disease Control and Prevention recommendations are that patients are no longer infectious after 7 days of illness and 3 days without symptoms.

Gaps in knowledge:

- Duration of shedding of infectious virus by recovered patients and the relationship to the detection of viral RNA.
- Knowledge of immune mechanisms responsible for virus clearance that might predict recovery and help determine when patients are no longer infectious.
- Immune correlates of protection.
- Duration of protective immunity.

APPENDIX

Authors and Reviewers of This Rapid Expert Consultation

This rapid expert consultation was prepared by staff of the National Academies of Sciences, Engineering, and Medicine, and members of the National Academies' Standing Committee on Emerging Infectious Diseases and 21st Century Health Threats: Peter Daszak, EcoHealth Alliance; Diane E. Griffin, Johns Hopkins Bloomberg School of Public Health; Kent E. Kester, Sanofi Pasteur; and Mark S. Smolinski, Ending Pandemics.

Harvey Fineberg, chair of the Standing Committee, approved this document. The following individuals served as reviewers: Kathryn M. Edwards, Vanderbilt University School of Medicine; James W. LeDuc, Galveston National Laboratory; and Steven M. Teutsch, University of California, Los Angeles. Bobbie A. Berkowitz, Columbia University School of Nursing, and Ellen Wright Clayton, Vanderbilt University Medical University, served as arbiters of this review on behalf of the National Academies' Report Review Committee and their Health and Medicine Division.